Dr. Messenger's Guide to Better Health

David L. Messenger, M.D.
with John C. Souter

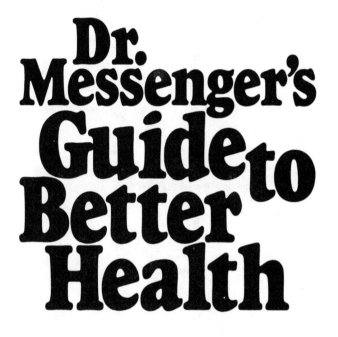

Dr. Messenger's Guide to Better Health

Fleming H. Revell Company
Old Tappan, New Jersey

Exercise Illustrations by Lavona Thomas

Library of Congress Cataloging in Publication Data

Messenger, David L
   Dr. Messenger's Guide to better health.

   Bibliography: p.
   1. Health.   2. Christian life—1960–
I. Souter, John C., joint author. II. Title.
III. Title: Guide to better health.
RA776.5.M47   613   80–20359
ISBN 0–8007–1113–0

To
my devoted wife
for thirty-three years
RUTHE

Contents

Appendixes

Preface

For the last few years, a number of patients have said to me, "You ought to write a book." Finally one of them, Bill Butler, became my agent and introduced me to my publisher, Fleming H. Revell Company. Having others feel the need for this book and receiving their encouragement has been beneficial in this task.

The title of this book was selected by the publisher. I would have preferred not to have my name in the title.

All of the information contained here has been learned from others: both from my patients and my colleagues in Wholistic Medicine. The concepts and ideas are not really new. I've had the opportunity to put them together in a little different way, but I can't make claim to any new or important discoveries.

Someday, someone may come up to me and say, "Dr. Messenger, your book has saved my life" (or something to that effect). Before that happens, I want to say that everything I know is something I've learned from the thousands of people who have touched my life. What is presented here is all a gift from others, so how can I say it is mine or take credit for it? As the sign in my office says: GOD HEALS, THE DOCTOR COLLECTS THE FEE. I have a deep sense of wonder, joy, and gratitude that I am able to be a part in helping patients (and readers of this book) have better health.

This book would not have been possible, if it had not been for the thousands of patients who have sought my help over the years. Many times I have gained insights and learned significant clues in treating people, just because they have learned to listen to their bodies.

I would like to point out there is a difference between "Wholistic" and "Holistic" Medicine. I believe *wholistic* is the proper term because we are to be "whole" people. Some use the term *holistic*, they say, based on the Bible's injunction to be "holy." However, biblical holiness is quite different from what these people are talking about when they use the term; in fact, many who use this term are involved in both cultic and occultic practices. I therefore feel that *Wholistic Medicine* is the proper name to describe my commitment to medicine for all of man's hurts.

My wife, Ruthe, has contributed much to this book. Most people who have eaten in our home would agree she is a gourmet cook. Her help has been invaluable in preparing chapters 5 and 6 on what to eat and how to prepare it. She's also put up with me through the years, as I've struggled with this project.

My daughter, Mona, and my son, Tere—though they are now married and live away from home—suffered to a degree because my wife worked in my office as receptionist, nurse, and business manager, helping me develop my practice and many of the concepts of Wholistic Medicine.

I'm appreciative of my office staff: Carolyn, Judy, and Joyce for their patience, when I have run into a lengthy, difficult problem that has upset the office schedule and created late appointments for many people.

I'm also grateful to John Souter, my writer, because he has listened to my explanations of a highly technical subject and has helped me convert it into a form lay people can understand. I might add that, as we have gone through the writing process, his eating habits have changed dramatically and he has lost over twenty-five pounds.

I'm also grateful to my pastor, Dr. Robert H. Schuller, for offering to write the Foreword to this book.

I would like to thank the physicians and staff of Placentia-Linda Community Hospital for their patience over the past years, as I have often used the not-so-customary nutritional therapies along with the usual medical modalities.

DAVID L. MESSENGER, M.D.

Foreword

I have known Dr. David Messenger for many years. He is a member of my church and an elder on our church board. He and his family are close friends of me and my family.

David Messenger is a great doctor. He is a great, mature Christian. He is concerned about the whole person, and this book reflects that concern.

Read it with interest! Read it with an inquiring mind! Read it with close attention! Read it and find healing!

This book can change your life, as you learn about the wholeness of body, mind, and spirit.

I recommend it! I've been helped by it, and so will you.

ROBERT H. SCHULLER
Garden Grove, California

Introduction

Each new patient on my appointment schedule is a mystery. I may face a little baby with a high fever, or a grandmother, experiencing the slow process of dying. My next patient may be a teenager, trying to find himself in a drug-culture world, or a successful businessman with the ominous symptoms of a heart attack. Each patient, though he has a single problem, is still a whole human being. When he gets sick, he doesn't get sick in just one area; he gets sick all over. When I deal with the disease process, I cannot look at a person as having a single problem. Each patient is a whole human being, and I must consider that *wholeness* in both health and disease. This is what *Wholistic Medicine* is all about.

Every patient who comes to me has one basic need: he is saying, "Doctor, I don't want to hurt anymore." Whether he is experiencing physical pain or an emotional hurt, he wants care and advice to free himself of the hurting process.

One of the best ways of easing pain is to help a person come to know and accept, and be happy with himself *as he is* at that moment. Physicians cannot cure anything because there is no cure for life. Life is a fatal disease. But that does not mean there is "no hope."

Man's greatest need is to be loved. In love there is hope and healing. Treating a patient as only one who has a cold, or a gallbladder or a heart attack, isn't accepting him or her as a whole person. To care for a person as a whole being is more than just taking a temperature or a blood pressure, or giving a shot of penicillin and a prescription.

One of the best treatments I have for my patients is the therapy of listening. I find that listening to a patient talk out his feelings—letting him know I'm trying to understand his difficulties—helps tremendously in the healing process. Mental anguish, the sense of uncertainty and hopelessness are often relieved this way. To be a hearing, caring physician is as therapeutic and every bit as important to medicine as removing a diseased appendix.

This book has been written out of my experiences spanning twenty-five years of medical practice—but I don't pretend to have all of the answers. Every time I go to a Continuing Medical Education course, regardless of the subject, I hear statements such as, "We're really not sure about this"; or, "We used to think it worked this way, but now we know that was all wrong." Medicine is a very incomplete science.

I believe this book should be just one in your arsenal of volumes designed to help you help yourself to have optimum health. Some subjects in it will not pertain to you; hopefully a substantial part will. It should not be the only book on this subject you read. Scan as many on the various aspects of good health as you can, but don't take any book as the "full gospel" on this subject. None of us has all the answers. Accept what fits for you, but don't worry about what doesn't. Sometimes, what is beneficial for others will be negative for you. That's the way life is.

This book deals with a variety of subjects, all designed to help you learn how to stop hurting and feel good. It's my hope it will improve the quality of your life. My goal as a medical doctor, a nutritionist, and a Christian is to help you learn how to have better health and peace of mind.

I
The Problem

1
"Doctor, I Don't Want to Hurt Anymore!"

It was after midnight, when I pulled myself out of bed and drove to the hospital emergency room.

The woman I was about to see was not my patient. A physician in a distant city had asked me to see her. She had become a nervous wreck—completely unable to cope with life.

My doctor friend had informed me she had a long history of mental and emotional problems. Over the past ten years, she had consulted a number of physicians but had found little relief. Even a year of psychiatric counseling had been of no benefit.

As I entered the curtained cubicle in the emergency room, I found a very distraught woman perched on the edge of the examining table. Her husband stood at her side, anxious and confused. His day had been long and frustrating, trying to console and comfort his wife.

After introducing myself, I commented, "You really don't feel good, do you?"

"No, Doctor, I really don't," she answered dejectedly. "I'm so tired; I'm getting weaker and weaker. I just don't have any energy. I can't even keep up with my housework anymore. This depression and anxiety has gotten to the point where I don't care about living. I feel so guilty, because I can't do what I should as a wife and mother."

She was the picture of despair. "My mind is so confused, I can't make any decisions. It's been almost two weeks since I've had more than two or three hours of sleep at night. I'm so worn-out I can't even stop crying."

Everyone Wants to Feel Good

Everyone who comes to me is saying, in essence, "Doctor, I don't want to feel bad. I don't want to hurt, I just want to feel good." People come to me because they are in pain and don't know what to do about it. I've been a practicing physician for twenty-five years and try to treat the "whole" person.

This particular woman was stressed beyond her ability to cope. She had passed her breaking point. Because a mental-emotional breakdown can often be caused by an overwhelming experience, I asked, "Have you had a major upheaval in your life recently? Perhaps the death of a close friend, the loss of a loved one—perhaps a financial calamity?"

"No," she replied thoughtfully, "not that I can think of."

I turned to her husband. "Your wife's problem is one we in preventive and nutritional medicine are seeing frequently. Much of my practice involves caring for similar illnesses. Only recently medical research has come to realize that in every illness there is a negative chemical reaction and/or chemical imbalance.

"I suspect your wife's basic problem is a chemical imbalance and/or toxic-allergic reaction within her body. I suspect a number of food allergies are the major part of her lack of energy, depression, and inability to cope. I recommend you permit me to admit her to this hospital. I will place her on a medically supported fast for four days. Then I will work out a program to selectively test her for food allergies."

I admitted her to the hospital, and on the fourth day of her fast, when I went to see her, she was a changed person—bright and cheerful. Her whole disposition had improved.

"Doctor, I'm so amazed! I haven't felt this good in months." Her eyes sparkled as we talked.

I began her food-testing regimen, and she proved to be allergic to numerous foods. Many of her favorite foods triggered the extreme physical and emotional symptoms she had been experiencing over the years. She was sent home with new knowledge about the effects of diet on her mental, emotional, and physical health. Over the next few months, as she watched her eating habits carefully, she began to feel better and better. Today she is a healthy wife, mother, and homemaker.

A Hurt Is a Hurt

A hurt is a hurt and a pain is a pain. We feel what we feel. No one can tell us what we *are* or *are not* experiencing. Recent research in neurobiochemistry indicates that all physical and emotional feelings are experienced through chemical reactions in the brain. Anxiety, hallucinations, anger, hot flashes, panic, and worry all have a physical-chemical component. Emotional feelings, such as bitterness, hatred, and resentment, though they may be triggered by external hurts, still are a physical-chemical reaction in our brain cells.

Over the past years, many in the fields of psychology and psychiatry have said that if a person would just think right and quit hating his mother, life would be happy and peaceful. We're now learning that a high percentage of emotional problems are based on bad chemistry, not just bad attitudes. Many, many thousands of people have been told in a snide, ridiculing way, "It's all in your head. You have a mental problem. You're just a little bit crazy."

Just because the good doctor could not find the cause of your problem in his blood tests, X rays, CAT scans, and sonograms, he attributed your problem to some mystical negative force within you, and said, "Go see a psychiatrist." Fortunately, this "pure science" attitude on the part of some physicians is being eroded by many new discoveries in brain-cell chemistry.

It is estimated that in a few short years, most psychiatric disorders will be diagnosed by means of chemical tests. So take heart! There is a lot more to your bad feelings than an abused and impoverished childhood. There are *many* chemical causes for physical, mental, and emotional illness which you can learn to free yourself from. People mistakenly assume such problems are all mental, when in reality these "hurts" are very often physical in cause and correction.

Helping the Body Help Itself

About one hundred years ago, Dr. A. J. Still, the founder of the osteopathic branch of medicine, said, "The body has all the potential to cure its curable ills." We have all had the experience of getting well from the flu, a cut, or a bruise without any professional medical help. Spontaneous recovery has occurred in almost every known disease. The natural ability of the body to heal its injuries and conquer disease is tremendous. Even we physicians do not fully comprehend how the body heals itself.

Everybody gets tired, sick, and injured. How well and how rapidly we recover is determined by our state of health. How we respond physically, emotionally, mentally, and spiritually depends on the available energy resource we have at that particular time.

With a little knowledge, you can learn how to help your body recover from its pains and sicknesses. I have been asked to write this book to help you help yourself. Everyone wants to feel good. Everyone wants a long life. By following the principles of caring for the "whole person," you can improve your chances of having both good health and a long life.

Understanding Your Structure

To understand how to help your body heal itself, there are some basic things you must know about the body's structure. "The Lord God formed man of dust from the ground, breathed into his nostrils the breath of life, and man became a living being" (*see* Genesis 2:7).

We were first bodies. We were not souls flitting around in space, waiting for bodies to be conceived. No, God took the dust, chemicals from the ground, and breathed into them the breath of life. The physical came first. Our bodies are the foundation for what we are, and our physical structure determines how we must function.

Often someone will come to me and say, "Doctor, can you give me something for my nerves? My problem is with my emotions." This is a common misconception.

People assume you can treat an emotional problem as an isolated condition. But this is not the case. All mental, spiritual, emotional, and physical difficulties are interrelated. Because these problems are intangible, we miss the fact that every function of life is ultimately the product of a chemical process within the cells of the body. It's hard to realize the brain functions as a chemical factory. Tranquilizers, alcohol, heroin, LSD and other mind-altering substances demonstrate the basic chemical nature of the mind. Yet, we seldom stop to think of food as a multitude of chemicals which affect how we think and feel. Nutrition—what we put into our mouths—is the essence of getting the mind and body to function optimally.

How High Is Your Energy Level?

Once you realize the body is a chemical machine which needs the right food chemicals to make it run properly, you will realize what you eat is *all-important* to your health.

The vitality of the body is measured by its ability to function, whether it is to think or feel or move. *Energy* is the basis of all of life's functions. Without energy there is no life. All of the processes of life involve motion and energy. Whether it is digesting food or thinking, the body requires energy and motion to do those tasks.

God reveals that the foremost commandment is to "LOVE THE LORD YOUR GOD WITH ALL YOUR HEART, AND WITH ALL YOUR SOUL, AND WITH ALL YOUR MIND, AND WITH ALL YOUR STRENGTH" (Mark 12:30).

Strength implies energy and motion—health and vitality. The essence of "loving God" is to have sufficient strength to function properly.

Dis-ease or disease is the opponent of good health and energy. When you have a fever of 105 degrees you don't have the strength to actively love God or anyone else. You will be irritable and unable to fully love even yourself, because of your low energy level. In other words, God wants you to maintain your strength, so you can love Him, yourself, and others to your full potential.

But people still feel, "If I can just rev myself up and get motivated, I'll be okay." Everybody is looking for a magic healing of energy. We don't really want to face our problems and the reality of life as it is. We are content to pop a pep pill or some other stimulant to artificially increase our flow of energy.

If you don't have enough of even one of the fuel ingredients that make the body run, you slow down the whole process. When you don't have enough energy, depression and anxiety come easily.

With reduced energy, it is harder to make decisions. You become irritable; it's harder to cope with problems; you lose control easily; you feel guilty because you cannot think and do what you ought to do.

The Origin of Our Hurts

Every hurt we are confronted with in life comes from one of two sources. First, we have physically induced pain, such as a broken foot, a heart attack, or cancer. Second, we have mentally induced pain, such as anxiety, depression, bitterness, and phobias.

Most of us think of such problems as heart attacks, appendicitis, ulcers, and ingrown toenails as being purely physical problems. This is not true. Each of the diseases that affect the body have an emotional side. Consider the heart attack, for example. In every myocardial infarction there is a distinct fear of death—we all know this condition can be fatal. Such a traumatic physical hurt invariably upsets our plans. It forces us to miss, at least temporarily, many of the pleasurable life experiences we are counting on. A heart attack produces definite emotional problems.

Consider the hurt of a broken leg; it isn't just the fracture of the bone that causes pain. On the emotional side, there is the disturbance of our plans by forced inactivity. We suffer being temporarily lamed. We're inconvenienced and can't do all the things we would like. We assume, "It will never happen to me," and when it does, we find we have powerful emotional hurts to deal with as well.

Even a flu episode can cause intense emotional suffering. When we ache all over, we become irritable, grouchy, and miserable. We feel guilty because we're not out there working. We have to become dependent on other people, which assaults our sense of independence.

Do you get the point? There are simply no physical-physical hurts by themselves. Every physical problem has its emotional side. The body and the psyche are intricately related.

The Cause of Emotional Problems

On the other side of the coin are the mentally induced problems. Fear, hatred, bitterness, anger, hostility, resentment, a sense of rejection, a sense of being exploited and betrayed—are all emotional factors. They are also symptoms of a spiritual problem in our lives. Just as all physical problems have an emotional side, all emotional problems have a spiritual side.

Why do I call these "emotional-spiritual" hurts? There are physical laws that govern the universe—such as the laws of gravity and magnetism. There are also spiritual laws that man must live by. If you violate a spiritual law, you will hurt because of it, in the same way you would if you jumped out of an airplane without a parachute. That isn't a concept or idea which I have thought into being; it's just recognizing and observing a universal principle.

How do we know there are spiritual laws? To answer, we must go back to the source of our authority. In the physical world we perceive through our senses. Because of the evidence we receive through sight, hearing, touch, and smell, we accept certain laws as being true, like gravity. When we go to the ultimate in spiritual law, the Bible, we find it is the final end point in the truths of spiritual law. Acceptance or denial of those laws does not change their existence.

In the very beginning, in the Garden of Eden, Adam and Eve, on being tempted, first doubted, then disobeyed God's law. Out of that disobedience came a sense of their guilt. Out of guilt came a feeling of fear. When God called, "Adam, where are you?" he responded, "We're hiding because we're afraid." Here we have the original sequence: doubt, then disobedience, then guilt, followed by fear.

As a physician, it has been my experience that when a person violates God's laws, he suffers, because of this willfulness. Lying, stealing, hating, lusting, and so forth, all result in negative emotional-spiritual hurting consequences in a person's life. As I will discuss in chapter 11, there is a chemistry—a negative chemistry—involved in each of these negative emotions. There is also a spiritual factor in each of these negative feelings. That is why I believe there is a spiritual involvement in most, if not all, negative emotions.

So then, all our hurting really comes from two sources: physical-emotional problems and/or emotional-spiritual problems—or a combination of both. If you blame God for a physical problem, like cancer, you will create an additional emotional-spiritual problem, or you can have a bitterness, resentment, or hatred emotional-spiritual problem that reflects itself in the body as disease. Sometimes a stomach ulcer, hypertension, eczema, asthma, and rheumatoid arthritis are the result of these spiritual-emotional disturbances. These are the two basic sources for all our problems.

Where Do You Hurt?

My job is to find out how a patient really feels—where and how he hurts. As a doctor of Wholistic Medicine, I am interested in more than the outward physical symptoms. I want to determine the true cause of a patient's pain and disease. I ask questions designed to help him see his problems more clearly. People who come to me are often unable to define exactly how or why they don't feel well, but the right questions often help them to give the right answers.

One of my early patients was a young woman on parole from the county probation department for beating her infant son. It took a while to discover the cause of her quick temper and irritability. After completing a diet diary, she realized that eating sugar caused her to become uptight and irritable; it was after eating sweets that she would lose control of herself. She didn't really want to hurt her young son, but her sensitiveness to sugar triggered her brain into overreacting to minor irritations.

"Doctor," she told me after several months of being off sugar and other refined carbohydrates, "I just don't eat sugar anymore because it does such bad things to me." Initially, this woman had a difficult time accepting the concept that her behavior problem was based on a chemical-physical reaction. She did not realize her diet played such an important role in her emotional life.

When it comes to living, most of us do what comes naturally. But doing what comes naturally is not necessarily the best for us. Often we find that what we've been eating is actually quite bad for us. A faulty diet can cause severe physical symptoms for you even though it may have no adverse effect on others.

I remember a twenty-year-old woman who came to me with a seizure problem she had had since age twelve. She was experiencing convulsions two or three times a week. Her parents had frequently taken her for medical help. Because tests did not show anything pathologically wrong, the doctors concluded she was suffering from an emotional difficulty, rather than a truly organic brain-wave dysfunction.

The woman had some awareness of what was said by those

around her when she was having a seizure. The paramedics and hospital staff often made derogatory comments about her that caused severe emotional pain. She developed a poor self-image because the doctors kept telling her, "It's all in your head." She eventually began to feel guilty, because she was mentally unable to stop the convulsions.

This woman turned out to be highly sugar sensitive. After changing her diet and taking her off all sugar, the seizures completely stopped. She has not had even one convulsion in over five years. Her story is just one in many of those who have had physical problems but have been unable to find the physical factor causing them. Hers was a physical problem that caused severe emotional problems as well.

In this book, I will try to answer the questions you might ask if you were to come to my office as a patient. In turn, I will also ask you questions designed to help you understand why you don't feel good—questions to help you find out why you act, feel, think, and behave the way you do.

For twenty of my twenty-five years in the practice of medicine I have majored in this specialty of caring for the "whole person." I'm certain you will be surprised, as I share with you many of the insights I have learned over the past years. You may also be able to discover some of the sources of many of your own problems.

II
Dealing With the Physical Problems

2
Why Don't You Feel Good?

How long could you live without oxygen? Under average conditions only several minutes. How long could you survive without water? Maybe only a few days. How long could you live without food? Maybe a month or two.

All of these elements are *essential* to your health and well-being. Getting enough unpolluted oxygen and water is an increasingly difficult task, but getting enough of the right kinds of food is becoming an even more difficult problem.

Misconceptions About Nutrition

When it comes to nutrition, we have to include all the basics—protein, vitamins, minerals, enzymes, fats, and bulk and fiber. But it is impossible to determine if you are getting enough of each of these essential elements by the look or taste or texture of what you are eating.

One patient, a young mother, brought her baby in to be checked for a cold. I noticed the bottle the baby was carrying had a watery orange-colored fluid in it. When I asked about its contents, the mother replied, "Oh, that's orange pop."

"Why are you giving that to the baby?"

"Well, it's just like orange juice isn't it?"

This woman was quite surprised to learn there is a vast difference between an orange soft drink and pure orange juice.

Another patient said, "Some of the things I like, and which are especially good for me, are apple turnovers, jelly, and cherry pie." When I asked why she felt they were good, she commented, "Because they have fruit in them. Everyone knows fruit is good for you." What the patient didn't realize, of course, is that the overload of sugar and white flour she receives in such products provide extremely poor and unbalanced nutrition.

Still another patient told me, "I eat chocolate bars to keep up my energy. I know they don't hurt me, because I eat them fast." She felt because she was eating them fast and not enjoying their taste that they would not harm her nutritionally!

Most of us grow up with some very foggy thinking about nutrition. We still think of meat as protein, milk as calcium, potatoes as starch, raisins as iron, oranges as vitamin C, when actually all these foods have many ingredients in them. It takes a wide variety of whole, complex, nutritious foods to have optimum health.

Most people have the idea that beef is our only major source of protein. But muscle meats, as in steak and hamburger, are only one source of protein. Eggs, chicken, fish, soybeans, beans, corn, and many other foods are also good sources of protein.

Often, when I recommend that a patient abstain from milk and milk products for a while, they are alarmed. They immediately complain, "But doctor, how will I ever get the calcium I need?" Milk looks like calcium. It's white just like calcium powder. But milk isn't our only source of calcium. Most people never think of green vegetables as an excellent source of this needed mineral, because vegetables are not white like milk.

Are You Receiving Your "Daily Allowance"?

If you look on the labels of most processed foods, you will find a little chart that tells you how much of your "Recommended Daily Allowance" you will receive by taking an average serving of that product. There are several problems with these charts.

They lead us to the assumption that every human being is alike and has the same needs—that is, there must be a minimum daily amount of vitamins universally needed. But no two people are "average." We all have individual nutritional needs that vary widely depending on our age, health, heredity, occupation, sex, activity level, and so on.

These lists of numbers on packages tend to make us think we really know what amounts of the various nutrients are necessary to promote health. But medical science simply does not know everything there is to know about nutrition, good health, and disease. In fact, the study of nutrition is comparatively new. Researchers are constantly discovering new vitamins and new functions for some of the more well-known nutrients necessary for optimum function of the human system. Medical science simply does not have adequate information to establish nutritional standards for everyone individually.

Finally, we have somehow come to believe that, through listing vitamins and minerals on our packages, we can obtain everything we need from the food we take off the grocery shelf. I'm convinced, contrary to common belief, that the average American diet is not "well balanced" or "nutritionally adequate."

Our Depleted Food Sources

God created a wide variety of food with a built-in balance of essential nutrients. When we refine, process, and purify our food, we upset much of this natural balance. Often much of the minerals and vitamins is refined away and most of the bulk and fiber is lost.

It is essential for our bodies to have a significant amount of indigestible bulk to function properly. Bulk and fiber pass through the digestive tract without being chemically changed. This natural bulk promotes peristalsis or rhythmic contractions that push food through and out of the lower bowel. They give bulky substance and increased volume to the bowel contents.

Another negative example of what processing does is seen in the milling of whole wheat to white flour. The principal reason for this is to extend its shelf life. A whole kernel of wheat contains approximately thirty nutritional elements. Refining strips many of these essential ingredients away. Even the so-called enriched flour has returned only three or four of these nutrients.

Sugar is still another depleted food. It is labeled as "pure" on the package—and it is. It contains none of the essential minerals, vitamins, or nutrients necessary to support life that were found in its natural state. It is so "pure" it is used as a preservative in some foods. Whether it comes as raw sugar, brown sugar or in the white form, it is a grossly unbalanced food. It contains almost no nutritional value—other than pure calories—and Americans consume approximately 125 pounds of sugar every year per person.

We all know it is in soft drinks and candy bars, but most people don't know it is found in about 75 percent of all foods available in our grocery markets. According to studies done by *Consumer Reports*, such products as Betty Crocker Hamburger Helper for Lasagna is 23 percent sugar—nearly three times the amount found in Coca-Cola. Jell-O, which is advertised as a "light" dessert, contains 82 percent sugar in the dry state. Quaker 100 percent Natural Cereal is 23 percent sugar. Wishbone Russian Dressing contains 30 percent sugar.

When you read product labels, you'll notice many names for the same thing—sucrose, corn sugar, corn syrup, maltose or dextrose. It's all sugar, and it is often listed as one of the major ingredients in processed foods.

I have a book in my library that makes a strong connection between the consumption of sugar and criminal behavior. I've already mentioned the woman who was on parole for child abuse, who realized that sugar made her extremely irritable and quick-tempered. A few years ago, the sheriff's department brought a man into my office for a glucose-tolerance test. The man had been responsible for a long series of sex crimes and, ultimately, a murder.

Soon after he started his test, he began to complain of weird sensations: the floor began to roll in waves like an ocean. He became extremely irritable and uneasy. His initial friendliness turned into hostility and paranoia. He quickly recognized these distinct mood changes himself.

When I questioned him about his past, he said, "Now that I think of it, many of my problems came after I had eaten lots of candy." At times he would buy and eat a five-pound box of candy all by himself, in just a few hours. Sugar is not good for any of us nutritionally, but for some people it is an emotional and physical poison.

Why Do They Process Food?

Why is food processed, then, if it takes away so much of its essential value? A major reason is the distance from the food source (the farm) to the table. Since World War II, technology has enabled the food industry to confer on most of our foods a seemingly eternal life quality. The use of preservatives, freezing, drying, coloring, texturizing, and an unbelievable variety of "modern" processing techniques can prolong shelf life and keep food from spoiling. This processing and preserving of foods makes them much more profitable for the manufacturers than fresh, whole, nonprocessed food.

Because of the large shift in the population of our country, there is a much greater distance from the field to the table. There is no doubt we need to preserve and store our foods to some degree. So what is the price we pay for all of this processing, purifying, and preservation? When we change the taste, texture, and appearance of food, add preservatives, and eliminate those parts that will cause it to spoil, it becomes increasingly more difficult to maintain adequate nutrition from our average daily food intake.

The canning process kills major amounts of nutrients. The contents of the cans are heated to temperatures far above the boiling point, often causing great losses in nutritional quality. So does freezing and refreezing, which is quite common to many food storage and preparation processes.

The best way to process packaged frozen french fries for home use, according to USDA (U.S. Department of Agriculture) technologists who invented the process, is to immerse them in the solvent used for dry cleaning clothes. Doesn't that make you want to run out and buy a package right now?

To make food look acceptable, food processors often change its true appearance. Oranges are dyed orange. Apples are waxed. Meat is texturized and sprinkled with chemicals to keep it red. Bananas and tomatoes are picked green and gassed to help them ripen at the right time. Research shows that a fruit which ripens on the vine has more food value than one which is picked green and artificially ripened.

When it comes to commercial meat production, we discover that the motive of the industry is more meat—faster and cheaper and with more profit. This is the reason the animals are kept in closely confined yards, fed scientifically calculated diets, and are shot full of drugs to speed their growth and prevent disease. Most agricultural scientists are not very interested in improving the nutritional quality of the animals we consume. They are primarily interested in improving the profitability of the finished product.

Many chemicals used in the processing and preserving of foods cause toxic reactions in our bodies. Others tend to destroy certain of the nutrients in the foods they are supposed to preserve. If you drank a glass of certified raw milk, laced with cyanide, your body would receive in part, good nutrition, but the toxic effect of the cyanide would kill you. Our food is good only if it helps us. If there are additives which affect the body negatively, the food value may actually be neutralized by a toxic reaction.

We can say that additives, whether they are preservatives, dyes, texturizers or other substances, added for any reason, more often than not detract from the nutrient value of our food. If you can get the same meal without all these added chemicals, you will be better off.

Depleted and Contaminated Soil

There are other problems, which also subtract from the nutrient value of our food. Today, many of our grains and vegetables are grown on depleted soil—soil that has been replenished with unbalanced chemical fertilizers (which do not adequately replace all of the trace nutrients). Our foods end up "looking" the same but containing less and less of the essential nutrients. There is evidence that the protein quality of wheat is significantly less today than it was fifty or a hundred years ago.

Another problem we face is pesticide, herbicide, smog, and many other types of environmental pollutants. We hear a lot about biodegradability, the rate at which a toxic substance is broken down and destroyed by natural processes. Many poisons, such as DDT, have a very long life. Once used, they stay in the ground for many years and are absorbed back into plants. Such pesticides get into our food chain and end up being taken into our bodies. The problem with these poisons is that they tend to be stored in our fatty tissues, which includes bone marrow. They may stay with us for years and years causing a variety of health problems.

Is Your Food "Alive"?

There is a new awareness today that foods we eat must be "alive." Inert foods, that is, those not capable of reproducing, are lower in food value. Spoilability is often a good measure of aliveness of food. Even though you take a vegetable out of the ground and it isn't growing anymore, it is still a live food and is very spoilable. Meat is from a live source and will spoil quickly unless refrigerated. Dehydrated or dried foods are still considered"alive," as are leafy vegetables, carrots, beans, and lentils. Fertile eggs and seeds are the most alive of all foods.

Foods that have been heavily processed have very little "aliveness" left. Most processed foods have been treated to the point where they will not spoil easily. The more a food has been processed, the less nutritional value it possesses, the less of your daily needs will be supplied by it.

Do You Have a "Balanced Diet"?

Balance in your diet is critical. You must have just enough of all the essential nutrients. You can tolerate too much of some nutrients much easier than you can too little. With most water-soluble vitamins, the body can selectively use what it wants and discard the rest. This is particularly true of the B complexes and vitamin C. What is not needed is flushed away.

It is possible to get a toxic overload of some vitamins, particularly the fat-soluble ones: A, D, E, and K. The body stores them well in our fatty tissues. Minerals are also easily stored in the body. This includes the toxic minerals and heavy metals such as lead, arsenic, cadmium, mercury, and aluminum. They can become an overload in the body, causing strong negative effects in your chemistry. It is also possible to have too much of beneficial minerals, such as copper, iron, and selenium.

Then there are the deficiency diseases, which come from having too little of the essential minerals. Too little copper brings anemia. Too little zinc stunts growth and causes poor skin healing. Too little iodine causes thyroid-gland problems. The more our food is grown on depleted soils, is processed and preserved, the less of these nutrients get to us per pound of food.

If you want good health, you must have foods that have the

proper balance of all the essential nutrients. You don't have to understand all the individual ingredients or be a supernutritionist to eat well. If you focus on whole, natural-complex "alive foods," free of toxic chemicals, you can improve your health. When you look at food, ask yourself, "How close is this to the way God packaged it originally?"

The Energy Crisis

There are two major chemical reasons why we don't feel good. One, we are not getting adequate amounts of good nutrition to function properly; or, two, we are putting into our body substances which are toxic and inhibit the human mechanism from functioning as it should (like driving with your brakes on).

Energy tells the story. The end point of metabolism is the energy of life itself. We need to produce optimum nutrition for our energy system to work exactly right. When your automobile functions at 90 percent of its capacity, and you lose two miles per gallon— you probably don't worry about it too much. But when the car functions at 50 percent of its capacity and you get only ten miles per gallon, you become concerned. The same is true with your body "engine," when it is deprived of the nutrients necessary to produce energy and support life. But most of us don't worry about our diets until we start to hurt or malfunction in some way.

No one has unlimited energy. Everyone must stop and rest to let the body renew itself. If you are not supplying your body all the nutrients it needs to renew itself, you will suffer from low energy and disease, or at least discomfort. But remember, it's possible to give yourself a nutritional "tune-up."

I recently had a three-year-old child brought to me because he was extremely hyperactive. This youngster was all over my consulting room, as I was talking to his mother. After about thirty minues of constant activity, he practically collapsed. He reminded me of someone who had just had an epileptic seizure. His eyes sank back in his head, his complexion turned pale and dull, and he lay in his mother's arms in a cold, clammy daze. Because of his superhigh activity, he had completely exhausted himself. His mother informed me that this hyperactive behavior had been going on since the day she brought him home from the hospital. She could never remember a time when he had not been unusually active.

I took the child off yellow foods, milk, wheat, and all chemical additives and placed him on six vegetables a day and some basic supplements. I asked his mother to bring him back in ten days.

When they returned, it was immediately obvious that the child's activity level had quieted by at least 50 percent. "For the first time I can remember," the mother told me, "it doesn't take me three hours to get him to sleep at night. When I put him to bed now, he stays there and goes to sleep." She thought for a moment and added, "There was one exception. My husband took him to the movies and bought him a hot dog and coke. He was up three hours that night before I could get him to sleep."

I saw the boy again yesterday for his allergy shot. His mother commented that even his father is convinced now about the negative effects of his former diet. "I work three nights a week, and his dad has to fix his supper. He's finally willing to fix his special foods, because he has to put him to bed and he can really see the difference."

I find that often fathers don't see their children enough to see the difference good nutrition makes in the behavior of their children. Men also have a deep inner need to produce a faultless offspring. They often blindly deny obvious medical problems in their youngsters.

Another child, who was seven years old when his parents brought him to me, had been classified as mentally retarded. I took a hair test (which I use to determine mineral deficiencies, as well as to evaluate any mineral toxicities and/or poisons in his system). I instructed his parents to keep a diet diary. He needed many changes in his diet to be nutritionally balanced. I also put him on some basic nutritional supplements. At the end of one year, his school had reclassified him from mentally retarded to being just a slow learner. My sole accomplishment was to change his nutrition.

Learning to Read the Signs

Your body is an indicator. It is an oscilloscope of what is going on within you. Think of your body as being the greatest test instrument you have. Every problem you feel happens for a reason.

We need to come to grips with the fact that all of us have something wrong—somewhere. Even the most perfect specimen of humanity has chemical malfunctions of some sort. If we were perfect, we'd live forever. We'd be infinite. In all of us there's an aging process going on. We have a built-in time clock that is programmed to run down and out.

The next chapter will examine the basic symptoms I see every day in my practice. It will give you the opportunity to ask yourself questions, so you can better understand how and why you are hurting. When you know why you don't feel well, you should be able to do something about it.

3
Signs and Symptoms

The first questions I ask any new patient are, "How is it that you don't feel good? What is it that bothers you most? If I had the ability to touch and heal you of just one thing, what would it be?" I ask this of all patients, regardless of why they have come to me. This helps them to be able to define for me what it is that concerns them most.

The *one concern* or *worry* that bothers the patient the most, is the one that must be dealt with first. The patient may have a cancer that's causing no problems, but he may have an ingrown toenail that's extremely painful. He wants relief now. In order to care for the whole person, I must know every way and every place the patient doesn't feel good.

The Most Common Complaints

The most common answer I hear is "I just don't have any energy. I just don't have enough strength to push myself anymore. The only way I get anything done at home is to push, push, and push myself. Then I'm totally worn-out, and I can't do anything the rest of the day." *A lack of energy* is the primary physical problem that bothers the majority of people who come to see me for preventive medicine and nutritional counseling.

The second most common response I hear is "I feel depressed." This can come in various degrees. Some patients respond, "I'm so depressed, I just don't want to go on anymore." With others it is not as big a problem, but big enough to be a major concern. It is discouraging to feel tired and depressed all the time. Many of my patients feel life simply isn't worth living, because of their bouts with depression.

"Have you ever had any thoughts of harming yourself?" I then ask.

Many patients say that they have thought about it but would never really follow through. Occasionally, I have a patient who has made several attempts at taking his own life. Depression is the second major symptom I see in people who are chemically and nutritionally depleted. In fact, I have found that more depression comes from poor nutrition than any other cause. These people are trying to run their eight-cylinder engines on only enough gas to run four cylinders. It simply doesn't work in our mental engine any more than it would in your automobile.

The third most common symptom which people complain to me of is anxiety. They're uptight, tense, and anxious. They have a sense of worry. They say, "I'm just a very nervous person. I'm always uptight and tense. I have all these pressures in my life and I can't control them."

"Do you worry?" I ask.

"Oh, yes, I worry a lot."

"Do you worry about big things?"

"No. I only worry about little things that don't matter much. I get uptight and anxious about insignificant things that don't make any difference, and that really bugs me."

"Are you irritable? Are you quick to 'fly-off-the-handle'?"

"Oh, yes, I can get really mean. I yell and scream at the kids. I find at times I'm a real grouch. I don't mean to be, but I just can't control myself."

Most of the symptoms I've mentioned here are not constant feelings. They tend to be up and down. At times, a person's energy is up; then, a few hours later, it is completely gone. At times they get very depressed. They're much more anxious and tense; they're much more irritable. It is important to note that often these people can be fine in the morning but be experiencing all these symptoms in the afternoon—or vice versa.

Symptoms of the Autonomic Nervous System

I ask, "Do you get dizzy, light-headed? Have you ever passed out or fainted? Do you ever have hot flashes or the cold clammies? Do you ever get white and pallid in appearance? Do you have sweats and perspire excessively at times? Do you ever have a sense of the shakes or tremors? It may be either an inner feeling or a visible shaking. Does your heart ever seem to pound or flutter or beat too fast? Or do you have a sense of irregular or skipped beats?"

These problems are all related to the autonomic nervous system located in the base of the brain. This nervous system regulates the heart rate, the flow of blood, kidney functions, gastrointestinal functions, and all of the automatic functions of the body. They're performed without our conscious knowledge or control. Obviously, there is no way you could possibly control all the blood vessels in your body with your conscious mind. Just that task alone would so monopolize your brain, you wouldn't be able to do anything else. That's why your blood flow, your gastrointestinal system, your kidneys, and all the other systems are pretty much controlled automatically. The problems discussed above are imbalances and disturbances in our bodies, which are controlled by this part of the brain.

Mind Symptoms

How is your thinking? Do you ever feel your mind is confused or spaced out? Do you feel strange in the head? Is it often hard to think? Do you find at times it's hard to make decisions?"

"Yes," many patients say. "There are times when my mind just goes foggy, and I can't make a decision at all. My mind is so unclear; I feel disoriented, I just don't think right."

"How's your memory?" I ask.

"Well, there are times when it's very bad. I can't remember anything. I go from one room to the next and forget why I was going into that room. Often, I'm talking to somebody and halfway through the sentence I've forgotten what I was saying. I'm so forgetful of little things."

"How about your attention span?" I ask.

"Yes. I often have to reread things. I have to go over and over things, until they finally stick in my mind. My attention span is very short. It's so hard to concentrate and keep my mind on what I'm doing."

Another area that stressed-out people find difficult is their "interest in life." They comment, "I'm just not interested in anything anymore. I haven't worked on my hobbies or things I used to like to do for months. I feel very antisocial. I don't want to be around people. I feel as if I want to withdraw. I often feel guilty that I'm not up to doing what I should. I feel I'm not treating my family right."

The Digestive System

Next, I go to the digestive system. "Do you have any difficulty with your stomach? Do you have heartburn, indigestion, acid, belching? Do you ever wake up in the middle of the night with stomach discomfort?"

When it comes to digestion, there are two areas of concern. The first is "indigestion," which is a before-meals problem. Eating or drinking an antacid such as Maalox or Mylanta often relieves it. Indigestion is more related to nervous tension; stomach ulcers are primarily a mental-tension problem. The immediate treatment for indigestion is to reduce the emotional tension, the stomach spasms, and the hyperacidity in the stomach.

The second area I'm concerned about is "poor digestion." When the stomach does not produce enough hydrochloric acid and/or enzymes, food does not digest well. After eating even a normal-size meal, you have a sense of bloating, fullness and biliousness. You may sense a lot of abdominal gurgling and distention. Your clothes may suddenly fit too tightly .

If undigested food stays in the bowel too long, it tends to ferment. When it ferments, it forms gas which gives you this bloated feeling. The treatment of simple poor digestion is to take digestive enzymes and/or hydrochloric acid. This makes up for what the body isn't making itself because of the poor nutrition, disease, or the degenerative-aging process. I have several patients whose stomachs produce little or no digestive enzymes. They must take enzymes before every meal.

Another cause of poor digestion and a feeling of fullness in your stomach can be caused by a blockage due to scar tissue or a cancer.

Don't assume it's just poor digestion. If it persists any length of time —even a month or two—see your doctor.

Colon Problems

Next I ask, "How are your bowels? Do you have a good cleaning-out bowel movement every day?" It is normal to have a bowel movement once or twice a day. I don't believe it is healthy for a person to skip a day, other than on rare occasions. If you regularly skip a day or two, then in my opinion, your bowels aren't functioning properly.

There is strong evidence that constipation tends to be a significant factor in bowel cancer. If you are eating something that has a carcinogen (a cancer-forming substance), and it stays in your bowel for three days, instead of passing through in eighteen hours, then your chances of getting cancer of the colon are greatly increased. It is the same time principle as touching a hot stove. If you touch it for an instant you probably would not get burned. But if your hand stays in contact with the heat for three or four seconds, you would probably receive a bad burn.

When you were an infant, you had two or three bowel movements a day. But as you grew older, your colon began to need more bulk and fiber to function properly. However, your diet probably tended toward the bland, low-bulk, quick and easy, highly refined carbohydrate foods. Missing were the bulk, fiber, pectins, and mucins of whole complex foods necessary to help you have a good cleaning-out bowel movement every day.

Diarrhea is the opposite bowel problem. Some people tell me they have diarrhea two or three times a week. They may go six or seven times in one day, or it may last two or three days, or even a week, before it goes away.

Other patients have the problem of a soft, sticky, hard-to-clean stool. This type of bowel movement is a prime symptom of an allergic colon. Your colon can have hay fever (an allergic reaction), and secrete mucus, in the same way your nose does. When you are eating a food to which your colon is allergic, you will produce large amounts of mucus. This alkaline mucus is mixed throughout your stools. An alkaline stool tends to cause anal burning and irritation, even bleeding. This type of stool is also very sticky and hard to clean. This is a food allergy problem.

An important negative bowel symptom is the passing of blood in a bowel movement. If you ever have blood in your stools, you should have it evaluated by your family physician immediately. It could be a silent cancer in your lower bowel. It may not bleed again for five or six months or even a year, but by that time it may be too late. Most tumors and other problems of the colon occur in the lower colon or sigmoid. Most of these diseases can easily be seen by means of a sigmoidoscopy examination. A hemocult test is a simple and quite accurate test for blood in the stools.

Other Areas of Investigation

Next I question about the KUB system: the kidneys, ureters, and bladder. "Do you have any problem on urination? Do you have urgency? Do you have pain? Have you ever had blood or pus in the urine, cystitis, or kidney stones?"

When I'm talking to men, I always ask about their sex drive. Many times they admit it is not what they would like it to be. Poor male libido or sex drive is often caused by physical exhaustion, depression, and/or nutritional deficiencies. Women also often experience loss of libido because of these same physical problems. Treating these deficiency problems often brings the sex life back to what they would like it to be.

Next I check on the lungs. "Have you ever had any problem with bronchitis, wheezing, asthma, pleurisy, pneumonia, or any other kind of lung difficulty?"

Then I look at the upper respiratory tract, or URT. "Do you have or have you ever had hay fever, runny or stuffy nose, sneezing, post-nasal drip, or sinus problems?" If you have any of these symptoms on a continuing basis, even to a small degree, you probably have an allergy. A cold simply doesn't last forever. A continuation of these symptoms is almost always an indication of an allergy. Many colds start first with an allergy, then move into a secondary viral or bacterial infection.

Next I look at teeth and gums. "How are your teeth? Have you had a lot of cavities? Do you have dentures? Do you have a bloody toothbrush when you brush your teeth? Are your gums easily irritated? Do you often have a sore tongue or throat? Do you have a painful or clicking jaw joint?"

A sore tongue can be an indication of a vitamin deficiency. I just finished treating a woman with pellagra, which is a deficiency disease of the vitamin nicotinic acid. She had a brilliantly red, magenta-colored tongue. Pellagra has been known for centuries. Without treatment it has a progressive triad of symptoms: dementia, delirium, and death. This vitamin-deficiency disease, along with scurvy and beriberi, affected many thousands of sailors in the fourteenth, fifteenth, and sixteenth centuries. We don't often see this problem today, and this woman's family physician and three internists had not recognized the disease. I treated her with a potent, balanced B complex, and she improved dramatically within ten days.

Another symptom much more frequently seen in B complex deficiency is a brown, furry coating on the tongue. I see this often in patients with colds, the flu, or other infectious illnesses. Cigarette smokers often develop a brown-black furry tongue, which is symptomatic of their B complex deficiencies.

A chronic sore throat, laryngitis, or cough can be an ominous sign of a tumor of the throat, a chronic infection, or allergy. Cold sores or canker sores (fever blisters), are caused by a virus. Changes in body chemistry allow this infectious agent to invade and break down the body's immunity system. This problem is found when the body tends to be more on the acid side. Taking large amounts of vitamin C tends to increase acidity, aggravating the canker sore problem. Alkalinizing the body with four or five calcium lactate tablets four times a day for three or four days should help this illness.

Another treatment that can be used for canker sores in the mouth is acidophilus powder. Take an acidophilus capsule, pull it apart, and sprinkle the powder on your tongue. Use the powder as a mouthwash/gargle, then swallow it. Often this will relieve the pain in minutes. The only difference between cold sores on the lip and canker sores inside the mouth is their location. You can use the same treatment for them, as mentioned above. However, there are prescription drugs that contain cortisone in a sticky base that are helpful for sores outside the mouth.

The Eyes and Ears

It is important to know if the patient wears glasses or contacts. However, the eye symptoms I am most concerned about, from a nutritional point of view, are blurring of vision, especially when tired, also light sensitivity or photophobia. "Are bright lights bothersome or painful to you?" Many people with metabolic deficiencies have a sensitivity to light. They are not able to tolerate bright lights. Pain in the eyes is often a sign of a more serious medical problem such as glaucoma, a tumor, or other conditions.

Loss of hearing is important for me to know, but I find the two most common ear symptoms of metabolic deficiencies are ringing in the ears and noise sensitivity. Many metabolically deficient patients at times find even average noises are quite painful and irritating. I remember one hospital patient who was so sensitive to noise during her food allergy testing that a clock ticking ten feet away caused her great discomfort. She had to be transferred to a quiet private room.

Other Important Body Systems

The *central nervous system* is next on my list. "Have you ever been in a coma? Have you ever been knocked unconscious or had convulsions? Do you have headaches? How many kinds? Are they pounding or steady? Are they on one side of your head or both? Do they ever get so bad that you have to stop what you are doing and go lie down? What do you take for them?"

The *peripheral nervous system* deals with nerves and involves such disorders as sciatica, shingles, neuritis, poliomyelitis, and paresthesia or numbness. I find that patients who are hypoglycemic often have vague numbness or tingling sensations in various areas of their body.

Next is the *musculo-skeletal-joint system.* "Do you have muscle aches or cramping? Do you have leg cramps at night or pain in your legs from walking too far? Do you have a sense of stiffness especially when you wake up? Is it hard for you to get going in the morning? Do you have any joint swelling, redness or stiffness of any joint in your body?" (This will be dealt with more in the chapter on arthritis.)

Skin Problems

"Do you have a rash, hives, boils, eczema, or psoriasis?" If your skin problems are related to allergies, you may be able to improve or control the problem by changing your diet and taking nutritional supplements. I had a patient who had giant hives; I've seen him when his back was one huge hive. He has learned to control the problem by taking fifteen to twenty grams of vitamin C a day. A skin problem may also be your body's way of telling you something else is wrong. Pain is a symptom that says something is not right. Many times you can be your own diagnostician. If you eat strawberries and break out in hives, and you repeat the experiment six times, it doesn't take a Harvard internist to tell you there is a problem.

It is well known that at times a married woman who is having marital problems will break out with a rash on her finger around her wedding ring. The rash can and should be treated symptomatically with a cortisone cream, but ultimately the patient must come to face the reality that the rash is just a symptom of a deeper emotional problem. Other skin problems are purely physical, such as poison oak and scabies. If a skin problem is infectious, as is impetigo, you need to be treated by a doctor.

Heart and Circulation

"Have you ever had scarlet or rheumatic fever? Have you ever had a heart murmur? Does your heart ever seem to beat too fast, or do you ever have a sense of an irregular or pounding heart? Do you have chest pains? Have you ever had high or low blood pressure? How is your circulation? Do you feel it is good or poor? Are your legs and feet cold at times? Do you have any varicose veins or hemorrhoids?

"Do you bruise easily?" Easy bruising is often the lack of specific chemicals in the blood. This deficiency weakens the blood vessels and capillaries, so that they break and bleed into the subcutaneous tissues causing black-and-blue marks in the skin. Bruising may be related to a deficiency in vitamin C, rutin, and/or vitamin K. This is something that you should not try to treat yourself, especially if it persists. There may be a much deeper underlying problem, such as leukemia or a blood dyscrasia.

I also ask about the endocrine and/or glandular systems. "Have you ever had any trouble with your thyroid—either high or low? Any problems with your liver, pancreas, adrenals, ovaries, or testicles? Have you ever had any blood-sugar problem, such as diabetes or low blood sugar, or other problems, such as gout, menstrual irregularity or anemia?"

What Are "Your" Symptoms?

Now you may be thinking, as you have read the last few pages, "I don't really have any of those symptoms, so there is nothing the matter with me." But, remember, no one is perfect.

I recently visited a diabetic friend. (He's had a heart attack and a stroke and had to retire at fifty.) "How are you feeling?"

"Oh, just fine!" he replied, smiling. But I happen to know he wouldn't be considered "well" by any life insurance company or potential employer. His "automatic" social response is positive, but did he feel good? Not really.

Everybody has physical and emotional hurts. Our first response to a hurt is to deny it and withdraw. Self-honesty and self-acceptance are our most difficult tasks. We tend to want to keep all that negativeness bottled up inside of us. We would rather not expose that side of our life to others. But if you are hurting, "not thinking about it" is not going to solve the problem in any way. In the next few chapters we will begin to delve into some of the answers for these signs and symptoms. We'll talk about basic solutions to these physical and emotional hurts.

Many of the symptoms we have discussed here have to be handled by your family doctor or an internist. There is no way I can cover how to treat all the medical problems detailed in these chapters. Major medical problems, such as ulcers, colitis, cancer, and asthma, simply can't be dealt with adequately in a book of this sort. The reason I've included all this material is to give you a total scope of the major signs and symptoms your body uses to tell you *something is not right*. Listed below are most of the basic health questions I ask. You may want to review them to see if you have symptoms that should be dealt with.

Health Questions

1 What's your energy level? Good? Not very good? No energy at all?
2 Do you get depressed? How often? How depressed do you get? A little? Lots? The pits?
3 Are you anxious, tense, and uptight? A little or all the time?
4 Are you irritable, quick-tempered, or grouchy? A little? Quite a bit? Really bad?
5 How is your memory? Are you forgetful of little things? Do you forget what you were talking about often?
6 How is your thinking? Does your mind get confused at times? Is it hard to think? Is it hard to keep your mind on what you are doing?
7 Do you find it hard to cope? Is it difficult to make decisions at times?
8 Do you feel light-headed or dizzy? Do you feel you are going to faint at times?
9 Do you ever get a sense that either you or the room is spinning around?
10 How well do you sleep? Do you have trouble getting to sleep? Do you have trouble getting back to sleep if you wake up? Do you wake up tired? Do you have night panics or bad dreams?
11 Do you ever have a sense of panic or disorientation that comes on suddenly for no apparent reason?
12 Do you ever get a sense of tremors or shaking? Either internal or outer visible shaking?
13 Do you ever feel your heart is beating fast or fluttering? Do you have pounding, palpitations, or irregular heart beats?
14 Do you have "the sweats"? Do you perspire a lot, at times? Do you get flushes and/or the cold clammies?
15 Do you have headaches? How many different kinds? How debilitating are your headaches? (*See* "Headaches" chapter for detailed questions.)
16 Do you have any blurring of your vision, especially late in the day, or when you're tired? Does light hurt your eyes?
17 Do you have ringing in your ears at times? Are you ever sensitive to noises? Are they irritating and upsetting to you?
18 Do you ever have a sense of indigestion, heartburn, gas, belching, or stomach cramps? Immediately before or after meals?

19   Do you have a sense of bloating, fullness, gurgling in the abdomen after meals, or a sense that your food doesn't digest well?

20   Do you have a good cleaning-out bowel movement every day, or do you often skip a day?

21   Do you have diarrhea for any reason other than a flu or cold? A little or a lot? Have you ever had blood or mucus in your bowel movements?

22   Do you have frequency of urination or a sense of urgency when you go? Does it take you a long time to empty your bladder? Do you feel you don't completely empty it?

23   Do you have a loss of sex drive or libido?

24   Do you have any problems with your lungs, such as cough, wheezing, asthma, bronchitis, or pleurisy? Have you ever had pneumonia, emphysema, or other lung problems?

25   Do you have sinus, sneezing, stuffy nose, stopped-up nose, post-nasal drip, cough and phlegm, runny eyes? Do you have a chronic cough or sore throat?

26   Have you had many cavities and fillings in your teeth? Do your gums bleed, or are they sensitive?

27   Have you ever been knocked unconscious? Have you ever fainted, had convulsions, been in a coma, or been delirious?

28   Do you have any sense of skin numbness, tingling, or a crawling sensation?

29   Do you have sciatica, shingles, neuritis, or any other kind of nerve problem.

30   Do you have any stiffness of your joints? Do you have a rash, hives, or boils? Do you have skin sensitivity?

31   Do you have any heart problems? Irregular heartbeat? Murmurs? Heart attacks? Angina or heart pain?

32   Do you have poor circulation? Cold hands, cold feet, or just a sense of poor circulation?

33   Do you have any swelling of your legs, arms, or face?

34   Have you ever had trouble with your thyroid? With your liver? pancreas? adrenals? or any other glandular problems?

35   Have you ever had a nervous breakdown? Have you come close to it?

36   How do you feel about yourself? How good or bad is your self-image?

37   What was your deepest hurt or greatest disappointment?

38 When was your last resting vacation, in which you took at least two weeks to do nothing?
39 What do you do for fun?
40 What do you plan to do with the rest of your life?

4
Quick, Easy, Convenient, and Unplanned Diets

It is becoming increasingly difficult to get adequate nourishment from our food, and most of us are blissfully unaware of what foods we put into our mouths. Without realizing it, we deprive ourselves of the proper nutritional balance the body must have to function to its full potential. Why do we eat this way?

Stop for a moment and think about why you eat what you eat. There are basically five factors which determine your tastes and appetites. One, your past cultural training (from your parents); two, availability of food products; three, convenience; four, your income level; and five, propaganda from the food industry.

Your Eating Habits

Eating is something we grow up doing but thinking very little about. What we eat is definitely similar to what our parents ate. What they fed us, we came to adopt as our own. So often we think that the foods we eat are what everyone eats, but if you examine the diets of people around the world, you will find the diversity is amazing. However, few countries have diets with the quantities of refined, processed, and preserved foods which we Americans consume.

We eat primarily to please our taste buds. After a child has lived for a year or so, he develops a sweet tooth. He learns that some foods taste sweet and some don't. Many children hold out, refusing to eat what is set before them, so that they can make it to dessert. Often parents give in and allow their children to win, because they're fearful if they "don't eat something" they will get sick. It is actually better for a child to go hungry for a meal or two and learn to eat the right food, than to be pampered and allowed to develop a taste for junk food.

Almost all of us fall into the rut of eating foods we like and avoiding those we don't. We usually have very simple diets which do not provide the variety and balance necessary for proper nutrition. As I have said earlier, the foods which taste the best are usually the ones which have the greatest amount of fat and refined carbohydrates and the least nutritional value.

Part of the reason we eat so poorly is that we grab whatever is available. The shelves of the average market are crammed with these heavily processed junk foods. There really isn't as much choice as there should be. It is difficult to buy the whole balanced foods that were available at the country market fifty years ago. For those foods you now have to go to a specialty store, where prices are higher. That special trip is too much work for most of us.

Last summer my wife and I traveled in Eastern Europe where we found breads made of coarse ground flours. The loaves were brown with tough chewy crusts. It was difficult to tell day-old from week-old bread, even though no preservatives were used. None of the breads was wrapped; it came piled in wooden boxes. It is unfortunate we Americans have come so far from the natural whole-grained goodness of the proverbial "staff of life."

A major factor in our diets is our desire for convenience foods. We live in a time-saving age, and for the sake of convenience, we buy quick-and-easy products—TV dinners, instant breakfasts, instant mashed potatoes, and instant orange juice. Such foods are not very healthy. The more processing has gone on, the farther we are from the original food source, and the less nutritional value is present.

Your income level is another factor in the food you buy. Ironically, it has been discovered that those with the least to spend use most of their money to buy the "fast foods"—junk foods with the lowest amount of nutritional value.

If you have the money, you can purchase foods that are fresher and closer to their original sources. Unfortunately, we often skimp on our food budgets, when this is really the last area which should be compromised.

Propaganda From the Processors

We have been sold a bill of goods by the makers of many processed foods. The fifty largest food processors purchase a large percentage of TV advertising time and easily persuade us to buy their junk foods. An example is found in the breakfast cereal industry.

Kellogg's, General Foods, and General Mills control approximately 86 percent of the ready-to-eat cereal market. These companies spend tremendous amounts for commercials aimed at children. Whether they use a cuddly bear (peddling Post's Super Sugar Crisp), an adorable tiger (selling Kellogg's Frosted Flakes) or any of the other innumerable characters created to sell these presweetened cereals, the results are quite profitable. According to a Harvard Business School researcher's findings, when buying cereal, mothers yielded to the wishes of their children 88 percent of the time.

There is a profit-exploitation factor in the food industry. When companies get extremely large, profit becomes more important than service to the consumer. The food industry emphasis has shifted from whole, natural, staple foods to those with more convenience, better taste, appearance, and longer shelf life. Such products are more profitable—even though they are less nutritious.

The large food corporations are masters of marketing products that are tasty and eye-appealing, but horribly deficient in helping us obtain a balanced diet. They push potato chips and instant potatoes instead of whole potatoes, because there is more profit in the processed products.

In my opinion, the food industry should return to the ideal of being of service to people first, instead of placing profit first. There is nothing wrong with profit. But if a company's sole goal is to make money (that is, to show a profit for the stockholders), then I believe that motive is wrong.

We live in the day of huge corporations, whose apparent sole goal is to make more money. How much money is enough? The whole Madison Avenue approach is, I believe, ultimately selfishness. Sell your product at any cost—brainwash the consumer for profit. That's the opposite of Christ's way. Greed is a deceit of

Satan, and it will never satisfy. I maintain it is better to go broke than to be a disservice to and exploit your fellowman.

Are You Eating "Junk Food"?

When I ask a patient, "Are you eating bad foods?" Many will invariably answer, "No, I don't eat any bad foods." What the patient really means is, he is not eating strychnine or lead or spoiled food. "I thought *that* food was good for you" is a common comment from my patients, when I review their diet diaries and find they are eating many processed junk foods.

What exactly is "junk food"? A junk food is any kind of food in which a major portion of its nutrition has been processed, refined, and purified away. The two major examples of depleted foods are white flour (which is the major type of flour used in this country) and granulated white sugar. Any food product which contains significant amounts of these two substances would have to be considered a junk food and of little nutritional value to the body.

Probably the most-often eaten American meal consists of a hamburger, french fries, and a cola or malt. Americans consume 33 billion hamburgers a year. That's an average of three burgers per person per week. Because of the beef, the bread, the milk (in milk shakes), and the potatoes, most Americans feel they are receiving a good meal. But let's look at that meal for a moment.

White flour and sugar went into the bun. There is a large amount of fat in the hamburger patty, which has an extremely bad effect on the body. There is a lack of bulk and fiber. In a cola, you have a large amount of sugar and caffeine and, of course, dyes. In a milk shake or malt you have many calories; it is a heavily sugared drink. The nutritional value of a typical milk shake is much lower than a glass of whole milk, and milk is far from being a complete or ideal food. This typical American meal would definitely have to be considered an all "junk food" meal.

When General Foods or some other company talks about nutritional value, they are not telling lies. Their food products contain everything they claim. The problem is they don't tell you what their foods *don't* contain. Processed products, on the whole, do not contain all of the necessary ingredients for good health. Many of the ingredients in the original food, as found in nature, have been lost in preparation and preservation.

The nutritional value of a potato chip is almost nothing compared to a whole potato. If you cut a potato into a thin slice and hold it up to the light, you will see a thin rim about one-quarter-inch thick surrounding the more prominent center. The inside is starch, while the outside rim contains the eye or the life of the potato with most of the vitamins and minerals. Fifty percent of the nutritional value and much of the nutritional balance is found in that outer edge. When we eat a potato chip, we get an overload of starch and a deficiency of minerals and vitamins.

What About Variety?

The diet reviews of my patients reveal most people have a very limited menu. They tend to eat the same foods over and over, day in and day out. Such diets eventually and inevitably cause health problems. If you take milk, beef, wheat, eggs, and potatoes from the menu of the average household, you will have taken away a substantial part, perhaps 50 percent, of their food intake. Eating heavily in only two or three food groups means you are not going to get a wide enough variety to obtain the nutritional balance you need from your food.

With the exception of vegetarians, I seldom see people who have an adequate vegetable intake. Not one in a hundred people begins to approach the amount of vegetables they need. A broad intake of vegetables will help you get the trace minerals and vitamins you need.

Most of the time, I find people do not think ahead or plan their meals, even when they are at home. They get in the habit of buying certain foods because of their taste appeal, or out of habit. They get into nutritional ruts. Their diets have a minimum of variety.

People in an urban environment usually don't take their lunch to work. Consequently, they don't decide where they are going to eat until quarter to twelve. Then they go some place where they can get it quickly and easily, and rush back to work by quarter to one. They end up in a fast-food place, buying something to fill up their stomachs.

Along with this fast-food meal, it is common to drink a cup or two of coffee, a Coke, or have a candy bar for a little afternoon pickup. These artificially raise our sense of well-being. They cause a false, hyped-up, artificial level of energy.

Avoid Eating on the Run

Hopefully, you are beginning to understand how vitally important food is for your health. Begin now to think of yourself as your
number-one priority. It is more important to eat right, than it is to
be a slave to the company-production line. You must eat with purpose and not haphazardly. If eating correctly makes you feel better,
hurt less, and increases your productivity, then that's what is really
important. Ultimately the *quality of your life* depends on what you
feed your mind and how you feed your body. These two factors are
opposites, yet they are as equally important as the two rails of a
train track. Your quality of life depends upon what you choose to
put into it one way or the other.

When you begin the day, make certain you are not so tired in the
morning that you cannot get up early enough to have a good
breakfast. If you start off deficient in your stored-energy reserves,
your productivity will probably suffer all day long. Begin right.
Make the breakfast choices that will enable you to live well.

Many people struggle with the social stigma of "brown bagging"
it. One of the signs of affluence is to be able to go out to a nice restaurant for lunch. Our pride and sociability cause us to want to go
out to eat like everyone else. But are we subjecting ourselves to a
personal priority that puts our health and well-being way down on
our list of important activities? It is only when we place ourselves
as the highest priority on our priority list that we will be able to
reprogram our thinking to eat correctly. Then it won't make any
difference what the rest of the world is doing.

Most foods can be used in a "fix and carry your lunch" situation.
Roast beef, chicken, fish, vegetables, fruits, nuts—there are so
many foods that can be taken to work to give you variety for your
lunch. Think ahead about what you are going to eat. Don't wait
until the last minute to plan your meals. If you plan your lunches,
there is no limit to what you will be able to take to work. You can
eat like a gourmet.

Eating Out

When you go out to eat, try to find a restaurant that offers a wide
variety of good foods. Choose a place where you can be selective in
what you eat. Look over the menu and try to find the foods which

are not depleted. Stay away from all dishes containing white flour, sugar, white rice, cornstarch, sugar-based gelatin, and all the other refined carbohydrates.

We are pretty much at the mercy of the people who prepare the food, when we go to a restaurant to eat. Restaurants fix their food for taste-minded not health-minded people. In ordering your meal, ask for a baked potato instead of a potato mixed with a cream sauce. By ordering the baked potato, you have the whole potato, which you can use with a little butter, instead of the many processed dressings. It's better to eat the outside of the potato and leave the starchy center.

Many of the vegetables and some of the meats in restaurants are served with sauces. Ask them to hold the sauces. In this way, you can avoid flour gravies. Another way to to be selective is to order a la carte or ask for substitutions. Have your hamburger without the bun. Ask for cottage cheese instead of french fries. Take a salad instead of corn bread. If you order a la carte, get foods that are boiled or broiled.

Don't eat breaded or deep-fried foods. The fats and oils have been heated to very high temperatures (up to 400 degrees) and they stay that way all day. The hotter and longer a fat is used, the more carbonized and rancid it becomes; both are very unhealthy factors. French fries, onion rings, breaded chicken, shrimp, and fish sticks have all been exposed to these hot fats.

You can have a reasonable and healthy meal when you eat out, or you can have almost pure junk food—depending on what you order. It all begins with your thinking; it starts with what your concept of good food is. Having a large variety of foods is as essential as avoiding the highly processed products.

5
What's to Eat?

The Food Groups

The common approach to nutrition in our society is to place
foods into four categories. These groups are dairy foods, meats, veg-
etable-fruits, bread-cereals, and some add fats-oils as a fifth divi-
sion. The concept is that you should eat something from each group
at every meal.

I seldom mention these food groups in my dietary counseling,
because in following people's diet diaries, I find people can include
some of all these basic groups and still have a horribly unbalanced
diet. Often a person's dairy products are limited to milk; their meat
is limited to beef; their cereal is limited to wheat; their vegetables
are limited to corn, potatoes, green beans, and lettuce. This limited
diet does not give you the balance and variety essential to good
health.

The Importance of Balance

The body needs seven types of essential food chemicals to support life. They are water, carbohydrates, proteins, fats, minerals,
vitamins, and bulk. By "essential" I mean substances or chemicals
that cannot be manufactured in or converted from any other source
by the body; that is, they must be supplied from outside the body.

1   *Water* is about 55–60 percent of the body by weight; it is our
    most important and immediate need. The average body func-
    tions best on eight glasses of water a day. Water is really the
    body's only fluid need. Such drinks as milk, coffee, tea, sodas,
    and juices are not fluid needs; they are taste needs.
2   The second basic food need is found in *complex carbohydrates*,
    i.e., starches and sugars. These must be eaten whole, natural,
    and complex, rather than processed, purified, and re-

fined. Refined or "simple" carbohydrates, such as white flour, sugar, cornstarch and corn syrups, sugar gelatins, white rice, peeled potatoes, most processed cereals (dry and instant cooked), are grossly depleted foods. In their natural "complex" form, these are the energy foods that are the basis of all bodily functions. They are our best overall source of energy.

3 The next group is the *amino acids*, which are the building blocks of protein. These are the basic structural substances of the body. There are ten essential amino acids from which thirty other amino acids can usually be made within the body. Only ten of the forty amino acids found in the body are "essential". Essential means the human body is unable to manufacture these within itself. These ten essential acids must be taken into our bodies in sufficient quantities to maintain life. Protein has an all-or-none law. That means all ten of the amino acids must be present in their proper balance, at the same time, for synthesis of protein to occur. Eating six of the essential amino acids for breakfast and four for lunch will not sustain life.

4 The fourth group is the *fats and oils*. These substances are an essential part of cellular structure and metabolism. They are far less essential as an energy storage (that is, fat deposits). Fatty acids are the basic building blocks of all fats and oils. There are only two essential fatty acids, linolenic and linoleic acids.

5 The fifth group is *vitamins*. They function to assist (catalyze) biochemical reactions in cellular metabolism. Those that dissolve in water are the B complexes and vitamin C. They are not stored well in the body. Not having enough of certain vitamins can cause deficiency diseases, like scurvy, beriberi, and pellagra. A, D, E and K are fat soluble and store well.

6 The sixth group is the *minerals*, which are divided into two categories: macro- and micro-nutrient. The macro—those needed in large amounts in the body (more than four grams per adult)—are calcium, magnesium, potassium, sodium, phosphorus and chlorine. The micro-nutrients are iron, zinc, chromium, aluminum, copper, manganese, cobalt, selenium, iodine, sulphur, molybdenum, vanadium, silicone, and nickel. An important difference between the minerals and most vitamins is that their overuse may be directly toxic to the body. Many of the trace elements can become deadly poisons if overused. Many, like chromium and selenium, are needed only in minute

amounts. The toxic minerals are beryllium, cadmium, lead, and mercury

7   The seventh need is for *bulk*. This includes foods that provide pectin, fiber, cellulose, and mucins. They are necessary for good gastrointestinal-bowel functions and for good peristalsis in the elimination process.

Eating Guidelines

First, you need fluids. Water, of course, is the best way to obtain fluids. Other good fluids include "fresh" squeezed juices, herb teas, and clear sodas. Coffee and tea are permissible in small amounts, when other drinks are not available.

Second, you need whole natural-complex carbohydrates. You can get these nutrients best from fruits and berries (one or two servings a day), vegetables (five or six servings a day), and grains (one or two servings daily). You should eat at least a hundred varieties of vegetables in a year. At least half of your vegetables should be eaten raw. Eat nuts and seeds (but not fried in oil), and legumes (lentils, dry beans, garbanzos, peas, limas, and so forth).

Third, you need protein. Protein that comes from a living source is much more likely to be balanced. Vegetable sources of protein are less likely to contain the essential amino acids in their proper ratios, while the amino acids found in fish, fowl, or meat are more complete. Eggs are a well-balanced protein, because they contain all the amino acids essential to the life of the chick.

You can be more certain of obtaining a good balance if you mix various sources of protein. Eggs, nuts, seeds, grains, legumes, sprouted seeds, low-fat meats, fish, chicken, and turkey are the best sources of protein.

Fourth, fats and oils should be liquid at room temperature. They should be polyunsaturated and never "hydrogenated." Soy, corn, linseed, peanut, safflower, and sesame seed are the best oils.

Fifth and *sixth,* you need vitamins and minerals. These essential elements are found best in vegetables, fruits, whole grains, and nuts. Minerals, of course, come from the ground, and plants receive their nourishment from the soil, so they are one of your best sources of vitamins and minerals. I believe supplementation is necessary for everybody, since it is improbable anyone can obtain sufficient amounts of these life-sustaining essentials without supplementation. (See the section at the end of this chapter.)

Seven, you need adequate bulk. This can be obtained from whole grains, whole fruits, seeds, nuts, and vegetables (preferably raw).

Helping Your Digestion

Digestion begins in the mouth. When you eat, eat slowly and chew your food well. Chew each mouthful six to ten times. The quick, "chomp-chomp-swallow" approach, bypasses the first step of digestion. Saliva contains starch-digesting enzymes. Chewing grinds and mixes our food with saliva, so it can be more completely digested by the body. You can slow your eating by laying your fork down between each mouthful.

There are four basic types of digestive enzymes. The lipase enzymes are for fats, the proteases for protein, the amylases for starches, and the cellulases digest cellulose or fiber. A fifth factor in the stomach is hydrochloric acid. In order for digestion to take place, all of these enzymes and hydrochloric acid must be present. If you have a poor-digestion problem, it is probably due to a lack of enzymes. A digestive enzyme supplement that contains all four of the enzyme types will be of significant benefit. (Many digestant supplements do not include all four.) If you do not produce enough hydrochloric acid, taking the enzymes will not be enough to improve your digestion—you'll need to take a hydrochloric acid supplement as well.

There are two basic kinds of stomach problems. One is indigestion with symptoms that tend to come on before meals, such as acid, burning, belching, or upper abdominal discomfort. These symptoms are associated with gastritis, ulcers, diaphragmatic hernia, esophagitis, and nervous stomach.

The second is poor digestion. This is more of an after-meals problem. It is associated with a sense of bloating, heaviness, biliousness, and abdominal distention. Also with this problem, you often have a sense of gurgling in the stomach. This is caused by not having enough enzymes and/or hydrochloric acid to develop the proper acid medium to digest your foods.

I have several patients who have lost the ability to produce enough hydrochloric acid and enzymes for good digestion. They must take a digestant before every meal. If they don't, they will have a significant amount of distress.

If your food lies in your small intestine or large bowel for an extended period of time, it tends to ferment. One of the results of poor digestion is abdominal and rectal gas. The poorly digested fibrous cellulose components of your food are a major cause of this problem.

How to Buy Food

Do a little checking before you accept the propaganda the food industry throws at you. Many label their products as "natural," but what does that mean? If we talk about foods from a natural source, we can easily talk about sugar, white flour, or alcohol.

Coal tar is from a natural source, but I'm certain none of us would eat it as food. It is mined out of the ground and is not from a living source—at least not recently. Although I don't believe it is possible to have everything 100 percent natural and organic— that's the ideal we should strive for. Purchase your food in as natural a state as possible.

What you buy is determined by where you live, the size of your family, the amount of money you have to spend, and how well the advertisers have communicated their product. While you can purchase just about every type of food at a supermarket, that doesn't mean you are necessarily getting the best products there.

If you can buy fresh eggs from a chicken ranch, fresh vegetables and fruit from a roadside stand, or whole wheat bread directly from the bakery, by all means do so. Realize that the large supermarkets cannot get these particular food items to you as fast as the specialty roadside stand or local bakery. The fresher your foods, the more nutritional value they have.

Read the labels, so you can avoid products with sugar, preservatives, dyes, white processed flour, white rice, and gelatin desserts. If at all possible, go to a specialty-food shop or health-food store to find whole-grain pasta and bread products. Noodles made with whole wheat are more nourishing than those made with white flour. Make whole wheat pasta yourself—you'll love it!

The Vegetable Scene

Today, about 95 percent of all vegetable calories consumed are supplied by just thirty plants. This is unfortunate, when you consider that there are approximately eighty thousand edible plants in the world (twenty thousand in the USA alone). Biologically, there is safety in diversity. Try to eat as many kinds of foods as possible.

How many vegetables do you eat? Look at the following list and mentally survey how many different kinds you eat: Asparagus, bean sprouts, beets, broccoli, brussels sprouts, chicory, Chinese cabbage, carrots, cauliflower, celery, cucumbers, eggplant, green pepper, lima beans, pumpkin, legumes, collards, dandelion, endive, escarole, lettuce, parsley, radishes, watercress, spinach, turnips, turnip greens, kale, kohlrabi, navy beans, salsify, Swiss chard, savoy cabbage, red cabbage, corn, yam, sweet potato, mushrooms, onions, rhubarb, rutabaga, sauerkraut, string beans (yellow or green), hubbard squash, golden squash, summer squash, banana squash, zucchini, tomatoes, romaine, alfalfa sprouts, leek, chives, okra, beet greens, scallions, potatoes, parsnips, rice, and artichokes.

How many of these do you overuse? How many do you underuse? How many have you never used? Remember too, this is certainly not a complete list of the various vegetables that are available.

Check at a bookshop or health-food store for a good book on vegetables. You'll want to know how to cook them, how to eat them raw, how to sprout seeds, how to season them, and so on. To stretch your imagination, walk into the vegetable and fruit section of your market and note every item that you *aren't* using. Usually there are eight or ten vegetables that you have never purchased simply because you don't know what they are or how to fix them. It will take a little thought to increase the variety of your vegetable intake, but the benefit to your health is certainly worth the effort.

Meat and Poultry and Seafoods

Again, with meat, you should have as much variety in your diet as possible. Besides beef, try eating lamb, rabbit, chicken, goose, squab, Cornish hen, turkey, duck, and wild game. In the area of seafood, there is striped bass, cod, flounder, halibut, tuna, whiting, scallops, clams, lobster, shrimp, hard and soft crabs, red snapper, eels, pompano, sea bass, fluke, smelts, salmon, mussels, oysters, conches, shad, and fish roe.

The less fat you eat, the better. Different animals have different fat content in their bodies. Select the cut of meat carefully, because the various cuts have differing amounts of fat.

You should have more poultry and fish in your diet than you do red meats. There is less cholesterol in poultry and fish, and you receive less waste and more meat per pound than with the red meats. Poultry is also easier to digest. In red meats, the marbling is the white fat interspersed with the red protein. This cannot be cut away. With poultry and fowl, there is less fat and it can be cut away more easily. Poultry varieties include chickens, turkeys, game hens, ducks, pheasant—almost anything that has two legs and feathers.

Pork has a great deal more fat than other red meats; it is also harder to digest. There are some red meats that do not have as much marbling; these are the wild meats such as deer. The younger and leaner your meat, the better it is for you. Range-fed beef, although not as tender and tasty, has less fat and more minerals. When you buy red meats, look for those that are bright red in color; they are the freshest.

Probably the most nutritious of the animal meats are the organ and glandular meats such as liver, tripe, heart, kidney, sweetbreads, and brains. They are richer in minerals and amino acids than muscle meats. As much as is possible, avoid heavily preserved meats— the packaged luncheon meats, sausage, cured meats, bacon, wieners or hot dogs, and so forth.

Expand Your Use of Grains and Legumes

When we think of grain, we usually think of wheat and wheat products. If you'll read the label on foods made out of grains, you'll discover there is wheat in just about every bread and cereal type of food. Try to use other grains such as rye, flax, barley, white corn, yellow corn, brown rice (long and short grain), buckwheat groats, millet, and triticale wheat. The legumes, soybeans, lentils, chick peas, red, navy and all the other beans should be included in your diet for variety's sake.

It is beyond the scope of this book to give recipes and extensive suggestions as to the type of baking and dishes that can be made with the various grains and legumes. Go to your health-food store and purchase a cookbook or two on grains. They will tell you how to grind and fix them in bakery goods, salads, soups, and so forth.

If you depend on the supermarket and the bakeries to expand your use of grains, you won't get too far. The health-food store proprietor should be able to show you how to use the other grains in place of, or in combination with, wheat. As an example, pearl barley can be put in the blender until it is ground into a coarse flour. If you wish to use a grain as a vegetable, you can cook it in chicken broth until it's tender, then bake it with onions and seasoning. Stone grinding of your grains is preferable because it is ground at a lower temperature and the enzymes and the oils of the grains have not been dissipated. The flour will be a bit coarser but more healthy and flavorful.

The Exciting World of Fruit and Melons

Take a look at the following limited selection of common fruits and ask yourself how many kinds you have tried: golden apples, red apples, Northern Spy apples, Rome apples, Baldwin apples, Russets, Winesaps, Cortlands, apricots, bananas, blackberries, blueberries, raspberries, gooseberries, loganberries, mulberries, boysenberries, strawberries, cherries, cranberries, dates, grapefruits, grapes (many varieties), mangoes, cantaloupes, honeydews, watermelons, nectarines, oranges, papaya, Seckel pears, Bartlett pears, currants, figs, peaches, persimmons, pineapples, plums, prunes, raisins, rhubarb, tangerines, and mandarin oranges.

It is always better to buy fruit when it is in season. Out of season fresh fruits have to be shipped long distances. That means they are picked green and ripened artificially. When choosing fresh fruits, choose those that have good color and which are firm to the touch. Anything overripe will be soft and may already have lost some food value. In the frozen department, there are many fruits individually frozen without sugar. Again, read labels carefully to make certain you are receiving fruits processed without sugar. When purchasing canned fruit, be careful to buy only those canned without sugar syrup. Dried fruits are another way to go. With these products, look for the use of preservatives.

Whenever possible, eat the whole fruit for maximum vitamin, mineral, and fiber content. Some fruits can be eaten without peeling. The kernels of some fruit pits are edible and nutritious. The problem is the time to crack the pit and shell out the kernel. This is the life-reproducing element and the most nutritious part of the fruit. Unfortunately, many of these kernels and seeds taste bitter, and some are toxic.

Dairy Products

Milk is the first thing that comes to mind when we think of dairy products. But others are buttermilk, cream, heavy cream, half-and-half, regular butter, nonsalted butter, cottage cheese, various types of yogurt, ice cream, countless varieties of cheese, dried milk, and many other milk-base products.

In choosing cheese, avoid the soft, processed kind. These have many additives none of us need. The aged cheeses (Jack and Cheddar) and the hard, dry varieties, such as Parmesan, are much more nutritious. Some cheeses, such as blue and some Italian, are not good for people who are allergic to molds. Some have been dyed with orange and yellow coloring agents. These are hard on those who have a sensitivity to these dyes.

Eggs are also considered dairy products. The fresher the eggs, the more flavorful and the better they are for you. As far as the nutritional value is concerned, the color of the shell is unimportant. Fertile eggs are better but not essential. Hard- and soft-boiled and poached are the best ways to fix eggs. Raw eggs are quite hard to digest and lose food value when beaten up or blended.

Nuts and Seeds Are Good for You

There are many different nuts and seeds to choose from. Try hazel nuts, walnuts, Brazil nuts, almonds, pecans, peanuts, Spanish peanuts, Chinese chestnuts, butternuts, filberts, black walnuts, hickory nuts, cashews, macadamia nuts, sunflower seeds, sesame seeds, and pumpkin seeds.

Nuts come in many shapes, sizes, colors, and flavors. You can get them toasted, roasted, salted, unshelled, plain, and mixed. The best way to purchase nuts is to buy them still in their shells, if you are willing to crack your own. You can find them year-round in markets. If you don't care to crack the nuts yourself, you can always find fresh nutmeats at the market or specialty houses.

We prefer the plain, unroasted nuts and seeds. If you purchase nuts and seeds that have been roasted in oil and/or salted, you run a greater risk of receiving a spoiled product—and of course none of us need the extra salt. When you buy roasted nuts, look for the "dry roasted" types. Unrefrigerated fresh-shelled nuts and seeds tend to become rancid and spoiled because of the high oil content.

Nuts and seeds have a high protein value and are also a rich source of oils. If you like peanut butter, you can use raw peanuts and slightly roast them yourself. Put them through the blender, while adding a little peanut oil, and make your own homemade peanut butter. (This should be stored in the refrigerator.) Nuts and seeds can be incorporated into casserole dishes, sprinkled on top of salads as they are served, used as a side dish, or eaten as a snack.

Fostering Nutrition in Children

One of the most difficult tasks a parent has to teach his children is to eat properly. This will be especially difficult if your children have become accustomed to sugared cereals, fast-food meals, and highly sugared bakery products. Children learn by example. If we want to foster good nutrition, it is going to be up to us to put it in front of them; but it takes more than just putting the right food on their plates.

One parent, alone, cannot improve a family's nutrition very successfully. Both parents must know what good nutrition is and decide this is what they want for their children and themselves. Parents can't expect to have a double standard of expecting the children to have a certain diet, while they go out and "live it up" or sneak junk food in for themselves. Working together, both parents can cooperate and teach their children how to eat the right foods.

Generally, the wife carries the burden of bringing in the proper foods, because she usually does the shopping, plans and prepares the meals. Throw out both the sugar and the sugar bowl. You don't have to have sweet things to eat. You can learn to like many foods that aren't sweetened with refined carbohydrates.

If your children are still in the cradle, your task will be comparatively simple, since they are not used to processed products. It will be easy for you to introduce them to good foods. If they have grown to teenagers and have not incorporated good nutrition into their way of life, your task will be much more difficult, because they have lived in an atmosphere of poor nutrition all their lives. This will take a selling job, but even a teenager can understand that by avoiding refined carbohydrates and other depleted foods, he will have more energy, less skin problems, less sickness, a clearer mind, and a stronger body.

Have a counseling session with your kids. Explain the harm that junk foods cause; explain how much better it will be for them to have proper nutrition. Anyone can learn to "like" new foods. They can learn to enjoy munching on carrot or celery sticks in place of candy bars. They can learn to eat nuts and fruit instead of cookies, cake, and sweet rolls.

Breakfast can be a problem, if your children have learned to demand the sugared cereals. You can cook whole-grain and cracked-grain cereals and serve them with a little honey and milk and cinnamon. Adding fruit to the cereal should take the place of adding sugar or artificial sweeteners. There are puffed rice, whole grain granolas, shredded wheat, puffed corn, and many other prepared cereals that do not contain sugar or other refined carbohydrates. "Long-cook cereals" are better than the instant-cook variety because they are less processed. Eggs and vegetables should also be introduced to your children, as other breakfast possibilities.

Lunches can also be a problem. The lunches served at school usually provide few vegetables. Home-prepared lunches allow for much more nutritious variety. When they eat at their friends' houses, or are served refreshments at church, they will receive cookies and punch and other items that are definitely depleted. Train your children on a consistent basis. Help them identify "junk food" items and how to avoid them.

Most children of today have been "treated" to the quick and easy, tasty, junk-food snacks. They feel taste is better than nutrition. But there are a multitude of good snacks available. Nuts, celery and carrot sticks, any fruit in season, dried fruits like raisins and apricots, cheese, and leftover cold meats cut into strips are a few examples. Cut up the celery, carrot sticks, and fruit. Put them into containers in the refrigerator so they will be ready at snack time. And, of course, eliminate all junk snacks from your cupboard.

What should they drink? Purchase canned or frozen concentrate fruit juices that do not have sugar added. There are also many small sugar-free cans of fruit juice which make just the right-size drinks for children. And make certain you have plenty of good drinking water on hand—even if it means buying bottled water.

Once you go through your kitchen and remove all of those depleted food items, you will want to make it a habit to begin reading labels on everything you buy. *I cannot stress this enough.*

What to Do for Dessert

Train your taste buds to enjoy fresh fruit for dessert instead of those rich, sickeningly sweet pies and cakes. In eating fresh fruit, you have nature's dessert right in your hand. You have the bulk and natural sugars that are absorbed slowly into the bloodstream. If you eat rich pies and cakes and foods prepared with shortening, white flour, and white sugar, you take in more calories than your body needs and overload the metabolism process.

Other good dessert selections are whole-grained pastries made with honey, baked custard, baked apples, cheese, and nuts. In baking custards and apples you can use raisins and honey, the natural sweetener. One of the biggest problems with honey is that it is a bit thick and hard to dissolve easily. Honey does not have to be kept in the refrigerator and it will never spoil.

Recently we purchased a bottle of barley-malt sweetener. It has been processed into just the sweet part of the barley flour. It is a little difficult to dissolve but it is much sweeter than sugar. My wife recently made a gallon of homemade ice cream, sweetening it almost exclusively with the barley malt, and had to use only a teaspoon and a half.

What About Supplements?

It is my personal opinion that in the current state of agriculture, food industry, and nonrural living we have today, everybody needs supplements. What do I mean by supplements?

A supplement is a tablet, capsule, or powder that has a large amount of vitamins and minerals. It should preferably be in a full-balanced combination, taken once or twice a day. An exception to this are vitamins C, E, and A which are needed in such large amounts, it is impossible to make a multiple vitamin pill or capsule large enough to contain the dosages needed.

The only vitamins that can cause problems when used in excessive amounts (that I know of) are vitamins A, D, and E. These are fat-soluble vitamins and are stored in the fatty tissues of the body.

The other vitamins are water soluble and are flushed from your body through your kidneys. An exception to this rule is that certain vitamins are toxic to some people in excessive amounts. But that's a different problem from the one the average person faces. I have found only a few people who have had adverse reactions from taking vitamins. Many times people are allergic to the other materials in the pill, the "incipients" used in making the supplements.

You should have all the basic minerals on a daily basis, especially the micro-nutrients. The minimum government standards here are fairly adequate, unless you have a specific deficiency. If you are going to have surgery, or have a prostate problem, your need for zinc is markedly increased. In pregnancy, the need for calcium and zinc, magnesium and B_6 are greatly increased. Whole books have been written on this subject, and I suggest you purchase a good one that gives adequate information on the various nutrients, vitamins, and minerals, and what they do for the body.

I feel it is necessary for our vitamin and mineral supplements to come from a source that is not highly refined or heat-degenerated—one in which the balance in nature has not been altered. The B complex vitamins are an example. There are a number of different kinds of vitamin B, but often we find these vitamin supplements coming in a single-entity form with only one of the B vitamins present. This is not the way God packaged these nutrients in nature. Only in a specific deficiency disease should you use only one of these B complex supplements alone.

Coal tar is the source of many of our artificial vitamins. In my opinion, they do not have the value of vitamins obtained from true organic sources. Whenever possible, try to purchase vitamins that come from a living source, rather than an inorganic (nonliving) origin.

Vitamin C is a big exception to this rule. It would be impractical and just about impossible to take large amounts of vitamin C (that is, eight to ten grams a day on a daily basis, or thirty or forty in a disease state), all from a natural source. Crystalline vitamin C can be obtained from the Bronson Company of La Canada, California. This powdered form of vitamin C is the most efficient and economical way to take the vitamin. Vitamin C fine crystals in the neutralized sodium ascorbate form are probably better than the ascorbic acid unneutralized form. My wife uses these crystals on many foods to give them a tangy, lemony taste.

6
How to Prepare Your Food

How to Store Foods

The storing of whole foods is an attempt to preserve our life-sustaining nutrients for future use. Future use could be a matter of hours, or years, or any length of time in between. Fresh vegetables or fruits can be stored for quite some time in a refrigerated warehouse. However, once they are placed on the grocer's shelf, they have a comparatively short life span. Fresh, perishable foods can be preserved best by freezing, canning, and drying; or they can be artificially processed and preserved by chemical means to increase the shelf life.

Since all foods are perishable, you will want to carefully examine the ways in which your foods are stored and preserved. Pick the method that will save the most nutritional value. For this reason, I encourage you to avoid foods in which chemicals have been added to lengthen their shelf life. Fresh foods have the highest nutritional value. Frozen foods are next best, then dried, and then pickled or smoked. The canning method of preserving foods destroys more food value than the other methods of food preservation.

Once the foods you purchase reach your kitchen counter, you must decide how to store them at home. Fresh vegetables and fruits should be washed and stored in the refrigerator. They should be kept in plastic bags or covered containers to maintain their freshness and crispness. If a fruit is not entirely ripe when brought into your kitchen, you can keep it on the kitchen counter at room temperature, so it can finish ripening. Some vegetables do not do well in the refrigerator, such as, potatoes, onions, yams, and tomatoes.

Frozen foods should immediately be placed in your freezer. They should not be left to thaw and then be refrozen. Every time food passes through a freeze-thaw-freeze cycle, destruction of the cellular structure of the food occurs. In the freezing process the formation of ice crystals damages the cells.

As a food thaws and the ice crystals melt, the water-soluble vitamins and minerals leach out of the food. Also slow freezing and/or slow thawing of meats, fish, chicken, and meat containing prepared foods allows the bacterial count to multiply rapidly. This is a frequent factor in food poisoning.

The door of your freezer does not have as low a temperature as the deep interior. So place your most spoilable foods well into the freezer compartment. Use the door only for nuts, seeds, spices, dried foods, butter, frozen juices, and bread.

There is a steady loss of nutritional value during frozen food storage. You should not allow any of your frozen foods to be kept longer than a year. Even that is too long for many foods.

Fresh meat should be placed in the refrigerator immediately, even if you are going to use it in the next day or two. If not, put it in the freezer. Ground meat will stay fresh a shorter period of time than will a roast. Chicken spoils faster than beef.

Dairy products should be refrigerated immediately. When using milk at mealtimes, pour out what you are going to use and return the unused portion to the refrigerator. If milk is left to warm up, it will sour and spoil much more quickly. Again, don't keep milk in the door of the refrigerator but place it farther back in the interior.

When food is canned, there is a substantial loss of the heat-labile vitamins and minerals. You can taste that difference when you compare canned goods with foods that are fresh or frozen. The contents of canned foods are processed at temperatures far above the boiling point, and any form of heating, as a rule, causes loss of nutritional quality. For this reason, canned foods are less nutritious than either fresh or frozen.

After you have consumed part of the contents of a canned food, do not leave the leftovers in the can but store them in a glass or plastic container. Have a regular plan of identifying and dating foods in containers so you can use them before too much time goes by. The longer the item remains unused, the less value and taste appeal it will maintain.

How Often Should You Eat Which Food?

Our basic protein requirement is about sixty to eighty grams per day. This can be obtained in two protein servings a day. Our basic fatty acid needs are met very adequately in whole complex foods.

On the other hand, the complex carbohydrates—our energy foods—need to be supplied to the body in small amounts, frequently. As carbohydrates are stored in only minimal amounts, the body has a continuous need for these fuel foods. Large amounts of carbohydrates at a time, particularly refined carbohydrates, tend to force the body to store these calories as fat. So small amounts of complex carbohydrates, five or six times a day, are the ideal for the fuel needs.

Free yourself from the idea that you must have a traditional breakfast such as bacon or sausage and eggs, hash browns, toast, coffee, orange juice, hot cakes, and so on. It's been many years since we've had a traditional breakfast in our home. The idea of having vegetables for breakfast is a shock to most people. However, countless millions in other countries of the world eat foods for breakfast that we've never heard of.

One of my favorite breakfasts is made of a bed of raw sprouts (usually alfalfa), topped with some kind of stir-fried meat or poached eggs and cheese that has been melted over them. Another breakfast I like is composed of bean sprouts, which are a little larger and tougher, so they are stir-fried for about two minutes with diced breast of chicken, ham, or fish. I also like zucchini, green pepper, chard or spinach (barely wilted and steamed), on which are placed two poached eggs or meat.

Eating Your Food Raw

I like raw tomatoes with the skin. Apples, peaches, pears, and a number of other fruits can also be eaten unpeeled. Some vegetables, like carrots, can be eaten with the skins on, unless you have medical problems and have been placed on a bland diet by your physician. Eat your vegetables raw whenever possible, but scrub the skins well before eating. Chew these foods well as large chunks of these course fibrous materials may be irritating to the bowels. Some vegetables should not be eaten raw. These include green beans, okra, rutabaga, also known as yellow turnip.

How to Cook Your Food

Frying in oil or grease is one of the least desirable ways of preparing food. First, there is the addition of extra fat (despite what many advertisers claim), which you don't need; second, the food reaches a higher temperature (oil gets hotter than water), heat hardens the protein which makes it harder to digest; and third, the heat destroys more of the vitamins and minerals. You can cook as well by broiling and barbecuing. This way you will not have the extra fats. In broiling, the fat drips down to the pan below. In barbecuing, the fat drips through the grate onto the coals.

One of the best ways to cook is the Chinese stir-fry method. This is done with small pieces of meat, fresh vegetables, nuts and seeds all cooked in the same cooking utensil. The meat is cooked first in a nonstick pan at medium heat—it should cook quickly in about two minutes. Then the vegetables and other foods are added. These foods should be cooked at a higher temperature, but only enough to heat them well and take away the coarse rawness. They should hold their shape and color and still be crisp when they're ready. Don't cook them too long.

Food that is cooked at a high temperature, say 400 degrees, should only be cooked for a short time. Vegetables, fruits, and meats are better baked slower and longer at a lower temperature. They can be baked in the oven, either covered or uncovered. In order to save energy, entire meals can be prepared in your oven. In doing this, you want to discern which foods take longest to cook and place them in the oven first. Later, add those that take less time.

The majority of the vegetables in our home are cooked by steaming. My wife has a set of stainless steel cooking utensils that have a good water seal. She adds a tablespoon of water, puts in fresh vegetables, then places the pan on a burner. When the lid spins, she knows the pan is full of steam and she turns the heat down to the minimum to let it cook for about ten minutes. My wife prefers steaming to most other methods of cooking because it retains the color, texture, and taste of the vegetables.

Never overcook. Overcooking destroys vitamins and diminishes the mineral content. It breaks down protein, and greatly diminishes taste and texture as well. You do not want to overcook your foods because they become soft and mushy. It is beneficial for you to chew your foods well. Firm foods require more chewing and this stimulates the secretions of the mouth and the stomach, which contain enzymes that are essential for digestion. There is more usable bulk and fiber in undercooked foods than in overcooked foods.

It is much better to steam your foods than to boil them. If you boil your foods, save the water and use it in juice or soups, it will contain many of the nutrients from the food. When you boil, food will never become hotter than 212 degrees. Foods cooked in a pressure cooker or deep-fat fried reach a much higher temperature and consequently lose more food value.

My wife never uses a pressure cooker, unless she runs into an emergency. If she sees that a roast is especially tough, she will hold dinner off for ten minutes and put it in a pressure cooker to tenderize it. Normally, vegetables do not do well in a pressure cooker. They come out with less flavor and are usually quite overdone. Frying, especially deep-fat frying, although a tasty way to prepare foods, tends to destroy much more of a food's nutritional value.

Barbecuing is another good cooking approach. Breads, vegetables, fruits, and meats can be cooked on the barbecue. Wrap some items in foil, such as ears of corn and potatoes. Vegetables and meat can be put on skewers and cooked shish-kebab style.

One of the newest methods of cooking is the microwave oven. The ovens come in all sizes and energy outputs. Be certain to check the market thoroughly before purchasing one. In the standard oven, food is heated from the outside in. In the microwave, heat is generated throughout, wherever moisture is present. The food appears to heat from the inside out. Different foods heat at different rates, depending on their water content. If you cook several foods at a time some items may overheat, while others remain uncooked.

Of course, the big advantage with the microwave is time. My wife especially likes her microwave for quickly thawing frozen foods. Don't try to cook vegetables in one of those plastic bags without penetrating the bag, or you are likely to have an explosion inside your oven.

Microwaves are fast and efficient for many foods. We like to poach eggs in the oven because the egg is done evenly, and you can watch through the door to see when it is cooked just right. In microwave cooking, the cooking process continues after the power is off, so do not cook too long. Some dry items, such as rice, whole wheat, grains, or beans will take just as long in the microwave as in the standard range, so you are really not saving any time on such foods. Also, remember you can burn foods in the microwave, just as on the stove.

Can You Still Bake?

Don't feel you are missing out on anything since you cannot use white flour, sugar, corn syrups, or cornstarch in your baking. You can still bake breads, cookies, pies, and cakes—only now you use a different approach. For refined flours and sugars, substitute natural products that will give your foods a greater richness.

It will take a little time to find the proper cookbooks and different recipes. You will need to experiment to determine what tastes good, but don't give up, because cookbooks *do* exist (*see* our list of suggested reading in the back of the book) and there are many tremendous recipes, using only natural ingredients.

Most people prefer home-baked bread to store-bought varieties. You can purchase whole wheat flour already ground, or buy a grinder and do it yourself. Some blenders, such as the Vitamix, are powerful enough to grind grains.

You will probably have to throw away most of your cake mixes, because they contain far too many processed items. Eliminate lard and shortening from baking and substitute butter, which adds much more flavor and is healthier. Substitute stone ground whole wheat and other whole-grain flours for processed white flour. Eliminate sugars and add date crystals, molasses, honey, or true maple syrup. These will add a different flavor, but you will probably find them to be much more palatable than sugar.

If you are going to use honey as a sweetener, you might want to keep some on your stove in a jar of warm water. When it is warm, it will dissolve easier and mix better in your batter or dough. Don't ever bring honey to a boil, because that will give it a strong unpleasant flavor.

When you use honey in baking, you must adjust your recipes. Use a little less fluid than the recipe calls for, and a little less honey than sugar, because honey is sweeter than sugar. To enjoy the use of honey as a sweetener, you will no doubt have to experiment, for there are many different varieties of this food substance. We prefer sage honey to sweeten our bakery goods, as it doesn't have a strong taste.

The Joy of Sprouting

Sprouts are an extremely economical source of enriched protein, vitamins, and minerals and are fun to grow. Almost any clear container that can be drained easily can be used. It is not necessary to grow them in the dark, and they can be washed and drained adequately on a working woman's schedule. You can purchase seeds from a health-food store or purchase the sprouts themselves. Eat them raw or add them to a wide variety of salads and other dishes.

Almost any viable seed will sprout under the proper conditions, but not all sprouts are edible. Potato and tomato sprouts are actually poisonous. Some of the seeds that sprout well and make tasty additions to your meals are: mung bean, soybean, lentils, peas, chick-peas, alfalfa or lucerne, fenugreek, wheat, barley, corn, flax, cress, lettuce, and celery. We've included a book in our list of suggested titles that will tell you more of the specifics about beginning your own sprouting.

What About Seasonings?

You can make exciting dishes out of dull foods that have not been your favorite foods by adding seasonings. When we think of seasonings, we think of herbs, spices, salts, peppers, and vinegars.

Seasoning salts come in many varieties and most contain sugar, MSG (monosodium glutamate), and other chemical ingredients. But you can mix your own. Start with sea salt and try adding any of the different spices and herbs in your cabinet. You might want to use a vegetable salt because it has less salt (sodium chloride) in it. Add small amounts of each item and write down exactly what and how much you have put in. Use the ingredients' label on a store brand of season salt as a guide in selecting the spices for your concoction. Avoid iodized salt unless you live in the "goiter belt" and never eat seafood.

Spices and herbs should be stored in a cool, unlighted area. If there is space in your refrigerator, that would be an ideal place to put them. Most herbs and spices have a shelf life of less than a year. The potency of the herbs is dissipated on exposure to heat, light, and air. Spices may become infested with insects, if they are not tightly sealed. This is particularly true of the peppers, paprikas, and chilis.

Another good seasoning agent is lemon juice. Sprinkled over almost any vegetable or meat, lemon juice will improve the flavor and perk up the taste buds. In lieu of lemon juice you can use vinegar. The best known vinegar is the apple cider type, followed by the white distilled and the seasoned vinegars with herbs.

My wife likes to buy vinegars in the gallon size. She will transfer some to a smaller container and add herbs from her garden. Try different herbs and see which you like best. If you don't grow an herb garden and can't purchase them fresh from your grocer, you can always use dry herbs as a substitute. Use sparingly, because in the vinegar a small amount of herb will produce a very strong flavor. Let the herbs marinate in the vinegar base for at least two or three days before you use your vinegar.

My wife also likes to make her own catsup and barbecue sauce, using pineapple juice as a sweetener. Try experimenting with tomatoes and come up with your own sauces. There are recipes for such items in natural foods cookbooks.

Party Suggestions

You are probably accustomed to serving cakes, pies, cookies, chips and dips, punches, and soft drinks—all products loaded with sugar, white flour, hardened oils and fats. What are you going to do to replace such goodies?

You can make punch with fruit juices. If it is necessary, these can be sweetened with honey. But there are many fruit juices that are sweet enough in their natural state. For carbonation, add soda water. (You might prefer to use fruit-juice concentrate and just add it to the unsweetened carbonated drinks. If it is too strong, add a little water.)

Dried fruits are another great way to satisfy the appetite at parties. They are easy to eat as finger foods and mix nicely with nuts and seeds.

We know a woman who took a cake-decorating class before getting into healthful nutrition. Now she owns all sorts of cake-decorating utensils and doesn't want to use them to make any of those depleted, sickening sweets. What should she do?

She can whip up potatoes and use some of the same cones for decorating around the platter containing vegetables or meats. She can prepare a stunning platter of food for a party, using all the techniques she discovered in the cake-decorating world and still present to her guests wholesome and delicious foods.

She can play with whipped cream around a large display of fresh fruits, decorating these fruits in many ways. Open some of the fruits, remove the pits and decorate the inside with whipped cream. The whipping cream can be sweetened with a bit of warm honey drizzled in at the proper moment. She can also make the white fluffy meringues for her pies and cakes with egg whites and a little honey.

7
The Diet Diary

Why a Diet Diary?

A diet diary is a daily record of everything you eat and drink. It provides an overview of what, when, and how you're eating. There isn't one person in a hundred who knows exactly what he's eating. In my experience, very few patients, even the nutritionally minded, adequately understand the problems in their diets.

When a patient completes a diet diary, it tells me the pattern of his eating. How many times a day does he eat? How often does he snack? How frequently does he eat a certain food? Does he skip meals? These are important pieces of information to determine if he is eating correctly.

I also look to see if a patient is overeating. There are two kinds of overeating. If you sit down and eat a whole watermelon, you make a pig of yourself and feel sick because of your overindulgence. But a second excess is far more damaging to your health, and that is consistently overeating one or more foods. If you eat six servings of wheat daily, or drink six glasses of milk each and every day—there is reason for concern. This kind of consistent overeating is harmful to nutritional balance. When you overeat one or more foods, you have to be undereating others. You probably will not be eating enough vegetables and other types of food to obtain sufficient variety.

Degenerative Diseases

Why is this important? Degenerative diseases involve the excessively rapid wearing out of the body tissues. A forty-two-year-old, who has hardening of the arteries and dies from a heart attack, is really missing his average life expectancy. His blood vessels have degenerated much sooner than they should have. The same can be said for a person who has a stroke at the age of fifty or fifty-five.

No one lives forever, but it is conceivable we should all be able to approach the average life span of seventy-three in a far-healthier state than we are. Any degenerative disease process which becomes clinically significant before we approach our life's expectancy is caused by too-rapid aging or degeneration. This happens because: (1) we were not endowed with healthy genes; (2) we have not provided our body with adequate amounts of the food substances it needs; (3) or, we have fed ourselves foreign food chemicals, which have been destructive to our body tissues. A diet diary will help you to be able to see how well you are (or are not) nourishing your body.

Are You Overeating, Undernourished, and Allergy Prone?

Overeating the same foods day in and day out tends to cause nutritional deficiencies. There are no perfect foods, and if we eat the same foods all the time, we exclude others, and soon end up with nutrient deficiencies. This tends to lower the body's immunity level and its ability to repair and regenerate itself. It tends to restrict our ability to cope with foreign substances—viruses, bacteria, toxic chemicals, and so forth.

Overeating one or more foods tends to increase the probability of developing an allergy in an allergy-prone person. Allergy proneness is a hereditary predisposition given to us in our genes. Some people are born with healthy immune systems, while others have marked immunologic weaknesses.

An allergy is a condition in which the body becomes sensitized to a specific foreign substance (a chemical that does not naturally occur in our bodies). This process takes time—it may take as little as five to ten weeks (once the sensitization process has begun) before the body will react in an allergic fashion.

The Different Kinds of Allergies

There are three different kinds of allergic reactions. First, there is the overwhelming, even lethal, anaphylactic reaction—a bee sting, aspirin, and penicillin allergies can produce such reactions. A hypersensitive allergic person can become violently ill within ten to fifteen minutes. Death can occur in as little as five minutes in some cases.

My wife had such a reaction to a bee sting. In ten minutes, she was covered from head to foot with hives. She was having difficulty breathing; her throat was closing up. Fortunately we were at home, and I had on hand an adrenaline injection which began to relieve her throat-closing problem. Then I ran every red light between my house and the hospital, literally praying for a patrolman to catch me.

The second kind of allergy is still very direct, but is a less severe reaction. You eat something and react within a short period of time. Examples of this are the asthmatic who begins to wheeze soon after eating peanuts; or the gasoline-sensitive person who becomes dizzy, light-headed, and mentally confused after breathing the volatile petro-chemical fumes. These are very direct, specific allergies.

One of my patients became quite violent whenever he inhaled gasoline fumes or paint fumes. After we discovered the cause of his problem he remarked. "Maybe that's why my mind always goes foggy when I use a felt-tipped pen."

Another patient had repeated bladder infections. When I was food testing her after a fast, she had a chemical allergic cystitis after eating an orange. Within thirty minutes she had bladder burning and discomfort. When another patient eats mangoes, her mouth swells, and she has a strong, burning irritation of the bladder within ten minutes. These are specific allergies that are fairly easy to detect.

The Hidden Addictive Allergy

The third form of allergic reaction is one of which most people are unaware. This we call an addictive allergy. This problem develops slowly over a long period of time. Smoking is probably the most familiar addictive allergy. Someone who is smoking two packs a day goes through withdrawal (a nicotine "fit") after six hours without a cigarette. Then when he smokes, he immediately feels a sense of satiety and relief. Why? Because he's feeding the craving or addiction.

Most people are unaware that you can become just as addicted to foods. Coffee is a good example. Many are literally addicted to it. One of my patients was drinking ten to twelve cups of coffee a day and as many Cokes. With this overstimulation of her energy system, she had exhausted herself to the point where she could not go on. While getting over her dependency and addiction to caffeine, she slept from fourteen to twenty hours a day for three weeks, before beginning to wake up and return to normal. I have had many patients go through significant withdrawal symptoms when they stopped consuming coffee, sugar, milk, eggs, colas, and many other addiction-producing items.

When we eat foods to which we have developed an allergic addiction, we get an immediate sense of satisfaction. Frequent use of a food we are addicted to tends to keep the dependency satisfied. It's only when we abstain from these foods for two to three weeks and then re-use them that we are able to detect the symptoms of the allergy. The longer we go in hours and/or days without the food, the greater the withdrawal symptoms will be. Then, after one to two weeks, as our bodies are freed from this addictive dependence, we begin to feel better and better.

Unfortunately, we eat so many different foods at a time, it is difficult to detect which food is making us feel bad. Also, we often think of foods in terms of their names, instead of their many ingredients. Unless you stop and think about all the ingredients in a food, it is difficult to pinpoint the chemical or basic food substance that is causing your allergy.

Let's take wheat as an example. Bread, pancakes, cookies, most cooked breakfast cereals, macaroni, spaghetti, breaded fish sticks, pie crust, cake—all contain wheat as a major ingredient. But we don't think of most of those products as wheat.

Milk is another example. Many of my patients say they never have milk, yet they eat cottage cheese, yogurt, cheese, ice cream, custards, and protein drinks. They consume multiple products made from milk.

Food allergies, then, come on slowly when we eat the same food over and over—constantly assaulting the body. People who have food allergies usually have multiples of them. They are moderately allergic to wheat and milk and beef and a list of fifteen or twenty other foods. All of these little allergies add up to a major allergy problem.

The Benefits of a Diet Diary

How can you determine if you are allergic to a food? How can you determine you are eating correctly? I believe the first step is to keep a diet diary. If for some reason I could choose only one diagnostic tool to work with, as a doctor, I would choose the diet diary. With it I am able to do more good for my patients than by any other single test I use.

Again, most people, even people who think that they are eating nutritiously, have very little awareness of what they eat. At least 50 percent of the people who keep diet diaries for me come back and say, "I didn't realize I was eating so poorly."

Many others think they have good eating habits. But these people often major heavily on three or four different health foods which constitute 50 to 70 percent of their food intake.

Wheat is good. Milk is good. Beef is good. But if you have an excessive amount of these foods in your diet, you cannot help but develop deficiencies. No food is perfect. If you are going to have a balanced, well-rounded, complete diet, you will have to eat a large variety of foods.

The diet diary is a teaching device. It helps you see the ruts you're in. You can use it to get more variety, bulk, and fiber into your menu; it will help you to cut out refined carbohydrates and other processed foods.

My beginning approach with a new patient, from a nutritional standpoint, is to first take a history (like that found in chapter 3). Then I order any tests I feel are necessary. I also have the patient keep a diet diary for seven to ten days. On the next visit, when I see the patient again, I review his diet diary and lab tests. Then I am able to help him with the problems he is having nutritionally.

But there's another side to the diet diary. It gives an opportunity for you to express how you feel (mood changes, physical symptoms, and so on) at specific times. Then you correlate the "what you are eating" with "what you are experiencing and/or feeling."

One asthma patient would wake up wheezing on certain mornings. As I reviewed her diet diary, I noted that each evening before an attack, she had eaten Roquefort dressing on her salad. I said, "It seems to me that this may be related to your asthma, because each time you've had an attack, you had Roquefort cheese the night before. Roquefort is a milk product but it is also moldy cheese."

"Oh, yes," she said, a bit sheepishly. "I'm allergic to molds." She was unable to correlate in her thinking that Roquefort cheese contains a mold. It wasn't until it was down on paper that she realized what was causing her asthma attacks.

Often, however, we have consumed a food for so long, we have no awareness of how it affects us. If, for example, you are allergic to milk (which you drink all the time), it will be difficult to discern. You may not hurt badly, but you do not feel super-good either. You might be suffering from a "low-grade" misery which you've grown into over a period of time. In this case, the diet diary can be used to spot those foods you eat to excess.

How to Use the Diet Diary

In Appendix A at the back of this book is a sample diet diary form. Copy the form, so you have enough sheets for a ten-day diary. Each day, write down the foods you eat and the fluids you drink at every meal, as well as snacks between meals. Be specific and complete; write down *everything.*

When you list a particular food, try to think in terms of its basic ingredients. If it is spaghetti, note that you are eating wheat, tomatoes, beef, mushrooms, seasoning, cheese, and so on.

There are also many "hidden" ingredients in the food. A common additive in bacon, ham, luncheon meats, and wieners are the nitrites. MSG, or monosodium glutamate, is a common ingredient in meat tenderizers, flavor enhancers, and many other foods. This last chemical is a frequent cause of mental-emotional and headache problems.

Another allergic problem I encounter is a sensitivity to iodine. Who thinks of iodine, when shaking the salt shaker? It doesn't say IODIZED SALT on the shaker, and you can't tell what foods it has been added to. But you are still getting it just the same. I am personally allergic to iodine and can't use iodized salt at all. There are also many kinds of seafood I cannot eat, because of their heavy iodine content. Look for and be aware of all chemical additives like these in your foods.

As you fill out your diet diary, listen to what your body is trying to tell you. Write down every symptom you feel in the space provided on the diet diary forms. Be sure to note the times you experience a headache, or stomach cramps, or mood changes, or drowsiness, or irritability. List every symptom that is not a good, happy, vibrant, healthy, energetic *you*. Doing this should make it much easier for you to correlate what symptoms go with what foods.

After you have kept your food diary for ten days, go over it carefully. Look for foods that are repeated often. I use a code—*B* for beef, *M* for milk and milk products, *V* for vegetables, *W* for wheat, *JF* for junk food, *RC* for refined carbohydratees, and so on. Or you can underline or circle each type of food with a different colored pen. This procedure will help you get the "big picture" about what you're eating; it will help you visualize the frequency of food use.

You will probably notice several foods you are eating in excess, and/or you may find one or two foods you suspect may be contributing to your headaches, depression, or some other problem. In either case, you will want to completely avoid those foods for a period of three weeks.

I'm not saying these foods are bad, such as "junk foods"; they may be whole natural foods that are causing your adverse symptoms or reactions. During these three weeks, avoid these foods (and also all junk foods); follow the suggestions in chapters 5 and 6 for eating well. Use large amounts of all the basic vitamins and mineral supplements to make up for any deficiencies you may have developed. When the three weeks are finished, you should have a food-test day (*see* chapter 8) for each of the foods you suspect are causing the problem.

A month after you've completed your food testing and begun to improve your diet, fill out a second diet diary. When my patients do this for me, I see how well they understand what I've been trying to teach them. This second diet diary and food testing, if necessary, will help you evaluate whether or not you have learned how to eat the right foods. Many times I do three or four or five diet diaries on a patient, at monthly intervals, to help him fully understand what a good balance is for his personal diet.

There isn't anything that's good for you in excess. Even too much oxygen is not good for you. I have a patient who is totally blind, because she was given too much oxygen as an infant.

It's even possible to drink too much water and get water toxicity. The son of one of my stroke patients gave his father sixteen eight-ounce glasses of water one day. The father went into a coma and almost died because of water toxicity. It was only as we went over all he had fed his invalid father that we were able to reconstruct the fact he had given him too much water.

You don't necessarily need a nutritionist to help you decide the foods that are bad for you. If your memory blurs and your head goes foggy; if you have fits of depression and feel bad all over—you *know* something's wrong. You know, because you're the one who's feeling it. All of these symptoms are chemical reactions. Learn to trust yourself and your symptoms.

One of my patients is so allergic to beef that one little beef-liver pill throws her into a depression that lasts for eight to ten hours. She had to learn to accept that just one little liver tablet could make her feel that bad for such a long period.

Why don't you begin work on your ten-day diet diary now? The only way you can begin to tell if you are having allergic reactions is to keep a written record of what you are eating and feeling. Then look for correlations between certain foods and your symptoms. The sooner you examine your eating patterns, the sooner you will be able to move ahead on the road to good health and free yourself from "dis-ease."

8
How to Fast and Food Test

Now that you have looked at your diet closely, what do you do with the knowledge you have gained about your eating habits? This chapter explains how to test yourself for allergic or adverse reactions to foods and fluids and introduces the principle of fasting.

Why Should You Fast?

If a normal, healthy person fasts, it will enhance his health. A one-day fast, two, three, or four times a month, is quite beneficial to the body. Fasting at least once a week has specific benefits to people with weight or other problems.

Some diabetics (and this *must* be supervised by a physician) benefit tremendously by fasting one or two days a week. I have even fasted diabetics who are on insulin. This must be very closely supervised and cannot be done if the patient has ketosis and/or is in coma.

It is my opinion, fasting should be an important part of most people's eating habits. There are two reasons for this. First, fasting will improve your health by allowing your digestive system to rest. Fasting also allows the body to rid itself of cellular debris and other toxic substances.

Second, fasting prepares your body for testing. I use a four-day rest and total fast to prepare my severely ill patients for a food-testing regimen. At least seven days must be dedicated to this procedure. I use this with people who have severe allergies and who are in a crashed-out state, as illustrated by the example in chapter 1. (This will be discussed later in the chapter.)

The Kinds of Fasts

There are basically two kinds of fasts. First, there is a juice fast, in which you drink a glass of diluted juice every hour or two in the course of the fasting period. This helps to keep your blood-sugar level up. It tends to avoid the dizziness, headaches, and the other withdrawal side effects of going completely without food.

Many hypoglycemics tell me, "Oh, I can't fast. I have to eat every two hours." That's not true. I have helped many hypoglycemics fast four days by using a juice-fast routine.

If you are going to use a juice fast in preparation for testing yourself for food allergies, you should use a juice you wouldn't use on a usual basis; avoid orange, grapefruit, pineapple, and apple juices. I would suggest grape, berry, papaya, and/or vegetable juices, such as carrot or green juices.

The second type of fasting is a total "water fast." Here you eat nothing at all, and drink only water for the fast period. A person who is accustomed to fasting, and goes two or three days without anything but water, should feel better and better every day.

The time factor in a one-day fast is very important. We are all aware we're on a twenty-four-hour biorhythm which we call the diurnal cycle. Your whole body metabolism, particularly the adrenal glands, is geared to this cycle. "Jet lag" is a disturbance in this twenty-four-hour cycle.

One of the worst things you can do nutritionally is to eat only once in twenty-four hours. Human metabolism is programmed for eating small amounts of food frequently, or no food at all. (Eating only once a day seems to cause the body to believe that food is scarce and it must store energy as fat, so it will not starve.) So, for a beginning fast, I believe it is best to go at least thirty hours.

How to Fast

The best routine for a "one-day fast" is to think ahead and plan a fast day. Have your normal breakfast and lunch. Then start either on water or juice. Skip dinner that night, breakfast, and lunch the following day. Eat the evening meal on the second day. This gets you past a twenty-four-hour cycle and away from food for approximately twenty-eight to thirty hours.

This schedule for fasting is also psychologically easier to handle. To miss dinner one night is not bad. The next day, you know that by 6:00 P.M. you can eat and you don't have to face another night of going to bed hungry. It gives you something to look forward to, which you would not have if you tried to go the entire day without food. However, some people who are not breakfast eaters do better by not eating from the evening meal and skipping all meals the next day and eating breakfast the following day.

After you have fasted one day a week for a while, you may want to fast two days in a row. But you must build up to it. Everything we do in the human body must be done gradually. For the average person to start out on a ten-day fast, as one man recommends, is pure utter nonsense, in my opinion. Psychologically and physiologically, that kind of abrupt fast could be particularly hazardous. It could also cause severe headaches, fainting, and so on.

Fast a day a week for three or four weeks, then try a two-day fast. If you can keep a two-day fast, then maybe you are ready to try a five-day abstinence. But plan ahead and build up to it. It doesn't make any more sense for you to try a ten-day fast as a beginner, than it would for you to get up from working behind a desk to run a marathon. The body is made to adjust gradually, over a period of time. It doesn't handle sudden jolts well at all.

Have a "Test Day"

The easiest way to determine if you have food allergies is to test yourself. Look over your diet diary and see if you can pick out foods that seem to correlate with your hurting symptoms. Once you have a suspicion which foods are causing your problems, you should completely avoid those foods for three or four weeks and then have a test day. (*See* Appendix B for Test Day forms.)

It is important you do your tests on a day when you can observe how your body is reacting. Don't plan it for an active, busy day, in which your mind will be concerned about other things. You will need to be sensitive to what's going on in your body, so you can determine whether you're having a reaction. Saturday, Sunday, or your day off are probably the best times.

Let's say you are interested in determining if you are allergic to milk. For your test day, you would drink two glasses of milk (and nothing else) for breakfast. Two hours later, eat a milk product like a large serving of cheese or yogurt. During this time, take your pulse hourly, just before drinking the milk, then every hour, until two hours after your last serving. You should carefully list any negative symptoms you experience on the Test Day forms, noting the time when those symptoms occur. When noon arrives, eat your regular lunch.

One patient recently completed a diet diary, then commented, "I'm beginning to think I'm allergic to eggs." As we reviewed his diet diary for the past ten days, every time he ate eggs, he had experienced a headache, light-headedness, dizziness, and depression. Sometimes these symptoms lasted a short time; sometimes they lasted all day. I took this patient off eggs for a period of time, and then had him do a Test Day with eggs. They were the cause of his symptoms.

Another patient, a thirteen-year-old boy, was taken off wheat and milk for a month. The boy began to fuss about milk, saying, "I like it and I want to try it." We used the simple Food Test approach on him, and had him drink two glasses of milk for breakfast before his next visit.

When he came in for his appointment he said, "Oh, boy, milk isn't for me. In twenty minutes my head was all stuffed up, my eyes were running, and I was wheezing from my asthma." He realized quickly, milk was something he could do without. If a thirteen-year-old can learn to read his body's symptoms, so can you.

The Seven-Day Fast and Food Test

If you are having extreme difficulties, you might consider the four-day fast, after which you will have a three or four-day food-testing period. The lady in the first chapter is an example of an extreme physical-emotional problem that needed to be diagnosed and treated quickly and thoroughly. With the seven-day fast and food-test program, we were able to significantly reduce the allergic reactions she was experiencing. Then in her food testing, when she ate an offensive food, her symptoms immediately returned.

In order to do a thorough fast and food-test program, it takes at least seven days completely devoted to the fast and testing procedure. It is not the kind of program that can be done while you are working or are active socially. It has to be done in a completely isolated situation. Again, let me stress this is not for the average person, but for that man or woman who is completely burned out—the person who has crashed and needs immediate help.

The purpose of a medically supported total water or juice fast is to take away from the allergic person all foods and fluids (and fumes) that might be causing allergic reactions. This gives the body an opportunity to be free of all allergenic food substances and to return to a somewhat normal state. (*Medically supported* means that all the basic vitamins and minerals are provided in therapeutic amounts in supplement form. This insures that the body will have everything it needs to make up for the deficiencies caused by the stress of the allergic person. It also means prescribing the indicated medications, as a temporary crutch, for sleeplessness, depression, and anxiety. They will help to bridge the gap and bring about a more rapid recovery.)

I would not advise you to start on a four-day fast *unless* you are in a controlled and supervised situation. One of my patients, a minister, was going through a severe bout of anxiety and depression. I suggested the seven-day "fast and food-testing" approach, but he was reluctant to go to the hospital. I agreed to let him try it at home, provided he would daily keep in touch with me.

In the middle of the night, on the third day of his fast, I received a frantic phone call from him. "I can't take this anymore," he said. "I'm having strong thoughts of suicide. I need help."

"Go to the hospital immediately," I told him. Once admitted, I gave him sedatives and started him on an intravenous feeding with supportive nutrients to relieve and control his hyperdepression and emotional instability. In twenty-four hours he was much improved. Then, as we began his food testing, it became obvious he was having severe reactions to quite a number of foods. Several of these food reactions caused his depression, anxiety, and suicidal thoughts to return.

After you have fasted for four days, you are ready to begin that advanced food-testing procedure. Let me stress again that this advanced food-testing program cannot adequately be done without fasting, because it frees your body from allergic reactions. Fasting is your withdrawal period.

When the body is being exposed several times a day to an addictive food substance, the symptoms are more or less constant. By avoidance of all food on a four-day fast, the body recovers to a degree. Then with a new exposure to the allergic substance, without the presence of any other foods, the symptoms will be much more definitive.

There are so many foods—which do you test? Use your diet diary to come up with a list of about twenty favorite foods—the foods you eat most often. You should test for milk and eggs and beef and wheat and any other food item you eat frequently.

Your allergy testing must be done with single foods. By *single*, I mean that food cannot be mixed with anything else. When you test for wheat, for example, use some pure form of the grain, such as a cooked wheat cereal. This way you will know that any reaction is caused by the wheat and not some other ingredient.

This will seem difficult and unpleasant to you, because you are used to adding milk and sugar and fruit to your cereal. But it is important to separate the food item you are testing from all other foods (except water). This is the only way you will be able to tell if you are getting a reaction. It takes longer for the body to react to grains, so you must have the grain three times in succession at two-hour intervals. (See what to look for in food testing in Appendix B.)

Using Your Pulse as a Test

Both in the Diet Diary (Appendix A) and the Test Day (Appendix B) forms at the end of this book, you'll notice there is a place to record your pulse and temperature. There are two purposes for checking your pulse. First, it can help you evaluate yourself for a possible thyroid deficiency, and second, it can reveal an allergic reaction more clearly.

There is a correlation between a low resting pulse and a low body-temperature metabolism. The low temperature (in the 96s and low 97s) and a slow pulse (50 to 60 in a nonathletic individual) indicate a low or slow metabolism, which is often related to thyroid-deficiency problems. It has been my experience that patients with a low temperature and slow pulse often feel much better on small doses of thyroid.

One sixty-five-year-old woman was totally unresponsive, she sat in a corner and stared at the wall in a mental fog all day long. She had been that way for eighteen months. Her retired husband had to take care of her every need. After correcting her diet and starting her on a small dose of thyroid, she began to respond and talk again. I gradually increased her thyroid medication till she was taking three grains a day. Over a period of eight to nine months she responded beautifully and became her old self again—happy, talkative, and doing all her household activities again.

The second reason for taking your pulse is to check for an allergic reaction. A change in a resting pulse rate (either up or down, but usually up) of more than 10 beats per minute, all other factors being equal indicates a reaction. The greater the change, the more significant the reaction. Before you test a food, take your pulse. Then eat the food and take your pulse again at one and two hours (or any time in between if you feel like your heart is pounding or fluttering or beating fast) to see if it has gone up or down.

How to Take Your Pulse

The usual pulse-taking site is the inside of the wrist, near the base of your thumb and just above the crease that separates your hand from your wrist. Bend your wrist slightly inward. Place one or two fingertips in the soft flesh between the radial wrist bone on the outside and the wrist tendons in the midline. Press gently until you can feel the pulse. Count for one full minute. If you cannot feel the pulse, try pressing either lighter or harder. Sometims the radial artery in the wrist is quite deep, sometimes it is on the surface. Often, moving your fingers, rolling or sliding the skin to a little different position will help you to feel the pulse better.

There are also two other sites where you can feel your pulse. The big carotid artery just below and behind the jaw bone and the temporal artery just in front of and above the ear.

Dr. Arthur F. Coca has written a book on the subject called *The Pulse Test* (Arc Books). The book will help you establish your average pulse. It teaches how to take your pulse before and after meals to check on the foods you eat. As it devotes almost two hundred pages to this subject, I will not go into detail here.

What Kind of Reactions to Expect?

When one of my patients ate anything with even a very, very small amount of sugar in it, his pulse dropped 20 beats a minute (from the 60s down to the 40s) and he would feel very bad and sluggish. Other people with allergies find the pulse becomes very rapid. It may jump from 70 to 100 or 120. An allergic reaction may also trigger an irregular heart beat. If on the seven-day fast and food test, you have not had a severe reaction two hours after you have eaten food, you can go on to test the next food on your list.

Be aware of any change going on within your body, no matter how small. It may be a headache, a sense of irritability, depression, dizziness, a stomach ache, shaking, and so on. You will have a tendency to blame reactions or symptoms on something in your environment. If you are in the middle of a food-test program and you receive a phone call which makes you angry and irritated, you will probably want to blame the caller rather than your chemical state of being hyperirritable at that moment.

Because you are so accustomed to thinking of your feelings as being totally separate from the body, that is, not caused by chemical means, you will have difficulty at first connecting these reaction feelings with the food you have just eaten. After all, the foods will be items which you were eating every day, and you will probably *not* have experienced such clear-cut reactions before.

One of my patients was quite stressed out. I put her through the hospital fast, and there was a remarkable change. In just four days, her moods and mental clarity had improved dramatically. I visited her after we began her food testing. She had just eaten some hard-boiled eggs thirty minutes earlier and had developed a state of marked irritability and anxiety. She was crying and defensive. At one point I thought she was going to hit me.

"But, doctor," she said, "I thought eggs were good for me." She ate eggs all the time. At home she would wake up and couldn't get back to sleep at night. So she would get up and fix herself an egg-nog. This drink would immediately make her feel better so she could go back to sleep.

This illustrates what we call an "addictive allergy." There is an immediate sense of satisfaction, pleasure, and ease. However, the secondary effects, which may occur anywhere from thirty minutes to two or three or ten hours later, will be negative mood changes and/or physical distress.

Another interesting occurrence with the fasting/food-testing program is a large weight loss. One of my patients weighed 144 pounds when she started. Four days later she was down to 132. She lost twelve pounds of water. Another quite heavy person lost eighteen pounds in four days. Allergic responses tend to make the body swell with water.

What If You Have a Reaction?

Let's say you have a significant reaction to milk or wheat or beef. Does this mean you will never be able to eat that food again? For the most part, if you avoid a food you are allergic to for six to eight months, you will lose much of your sensitivity. Often you can then go back to eating that food on an infrequent basis. Sometimes, however, these food allergies last for years.

I personally was allergic to oranges and grapefruit for over twenty years. I couldn't consume them, even in small amounts, without a distressing bowel reaction. In the past year I find I can tolerate citrus fruits once or twice a month, with no negative symptoms.

What I do with patients who have a multitude of food allergies is to put them on a rotation diet. They may eat a food they are aller-gic to only once in four or seven days. Usually the allergic sub-stance will stimulate only a mild reaction when it is eaten this in-frequently.

You may find one or two foods that you must completely abstain from. But once you have been away from the allergy-stimulating food for a period of time, you will *usually* be able to tolerate the food on an infrequent basis.

Skin tests, allergy shots, and nutritional therapy will be very helpful in this kind of problem. Over a long period of time, allergy shots may reduce one's susceptibility and reactions to many foods, pollens, and other inhalants. But for the acute reactions, however, avoidance is the best approach.

The allergic response to a food, such as beef or eggs, is due to the fact that beef and egg protein molecules are incompletely digested (that is, separated into individual amino acids components). The protein molecule is big enough to maintain its chemical identity. Such molecules are "foreign" to our chemistry, and thus our bodies react to them. By improving digestion through the use of all four of the digestive enzymes and/or hydrochloric acid, the foreign protein molecules are more completely broken down. The more completely a food is digested, the less foreign it is to our body chemistry. The less foreign it is, the less allergy reacting it is. Chapter 3 talks about digestion in greater detail.

You Can Feel Better

One of the most remarkable "turnarounds" in a food-allergic patient under my care was a fifty-year-old chronic alcoholic. He was paranoid, hostile, and irritable to the point where he and his family felt quite estranged. He had severe debilitating headaches and had attempted suicide before coming to me. He was desperate and ready to try anything, so I admitted him to the hospital and began the seven-day fast and food-testing procedure. In four days, the change in the man's behavior was clinically obvious to everyone.

When we began to test him, the food he showed the most remarkable reaction to was peanut butter. After we gave him a tablespoon of it, he immediately felt uncomfortable. In just a few minutes, he developed both audio and visual hallucinations. He began to hear voices, and to see flashes of light and weird shapes. Other foods also had similar effects on his mind. Before, when he had heard these voices at home and on the job, he thought people were talking about him. This caused him to become extremely paranoid, and he drank heavily. The food testing convinced him the hallucinations and the voices were inside his head, and were caused by food chemicals acting on his brain.

I instructed him to completely abstain from all the foods he was even slightly allergic to. Several months later he came in to see me. "Doctor, this is the first Christmas I can ever remember. This year I had a wonderful time with my children and grandchildren, because I wasn't drunk and hostile as in previous years."

A year later he came to see me again. He was off alcohol completely and had really learned to listen to his body. He could tell me the foods that made him hurt; he knew them well.

Another lady came to me with severe debilitating headaches. The pain was so distressing for this thirty-five-year-old woman, she could often not go to work. When we took her history she commented, "I remember having headaches when I was in first grade. Often I would not go out to play at recess because of my headaches."

After fasting in the hospital for four days, her headaches were gone. During the testing period, one of her food challenges was plain granulated sugar. Within minutes, she developed an intense, severe headache. I find more people are sensitive to sugar than any other food or additive.

A month after the testing, the woman came in to see me. "Doctor, I've only had one headache this entire month! This is the first time I can *ever* remember going so long without a headache!" The only time she had had a headache, she inadvertently ate a food which contained sugar. Sugar is hidden in so many foods, it is difficult to avoid it completely, but this woman learned even a little was like poison to her head.

9
A Physical Fitness Program

Ultimate body fitness is more than just food—it involves physical activity, emotional well-being, and adequate amounts of rest. I believe the first part of physical fitness is rest.

How's Your Energy Account?

Most of us are too busy with activities. The first thing I do for patients who have overworked themselves or "burned out" is to put them on sick leave or disability. Sometimes this is just for a few weeks; at other times it is for months. Their total body condition has become so stressed out they just don't have the energy to function properly.

I insist these people get plenty of rest, even if it means twelve, sixteen or twenty hours of sleep a day. We get so caught up in the hustle of living, we push ourselves, until we have used up all our energy reserve.

Each of us has two energy systems. One is like the checking account of our day-to-day expenses (or activities); the other is our savings account, where we store energy for those stressful or emergency times. When you spend more energy than is stored in your checking account, you must dip into your energy reserve, If you keep pushing yourself, eventually you won't have any reserve left, and your energy checks begin to bounce. This is why you end up weak, tired, fatigued, and worn-out.

The beginning of fitness is to rest enough, so your body can renew itself sufficiently to be active. You must have enough energy to carry out your daily activities, as well as a reserve for the extra stresses and pressures of life. I find most people are so programmed to activity that they feel guilty about doing nothing.

The Importance of Vacations

When was your last "get-away-and-rest" vacation? This is a very important question. "Well, we take weekends," many people tell me. The average person has many problems on his mind and feels pressured by the stress of family and business concerns. But we must learn to take time off! If God needed to rest on the seventh day, who do you think you are to work right through the weekend year in and year out? I have seen many executives burn themselves out just because they did not take vacations.

I remember one thirty-six-year-old fellow who told me, "Oh, I take long weekends and four-day holidays."

"No," I said. "When was your last two-week resting vacation?"

"I've been working for my company sixteen years and I've never taken a vacation." You could look at this man and tell he was burned out. His eyes had no sparkle. He had to think for some time about my questions before he could answer.

Some years ago I read how a large company on the East Coast had studied this problem. They found they had much more productivity out of their eleven-month work and one-month vacation employees than they did out of those who worked all twelve.

We get this superman complex and feel "only I" can do the job. So we keep pushing ourselves, until we go over the brink. Then we end up with a heart attack, or ulcers, or a nervous breakdown, or even suicide—all just because we didn't think enough of ourselves and our families to take a vacation.

If you were an automobile, we could overhaul your carburetor, give you a tune up, and put you back on the road—but, as a human being, it takes time for your body to renew itself and get back up to maximum efficiency.

I'm certain it takes a minimum of two weeks—preferably a month—of doing nothing, to give you the physical and mental rejuvenation you need. I really believe that's the only way to get your mind off your problems and the energy reserve back into your system. Four days here and there over the year is just not going to do it.

This comes back to self-confidence. You have to believe enough in yourself and what you've done to leave the job for a few weeks without being fearful things are going to fall apart. You have to believe you can get all your work done when you return. Vacations are absolutely important to your good health.

The Rest Cycle

You also need a rest cycle on the job. The best daily work plan I know of was devised by an artist, Walter Russell. This man worked two hours at painting, two hours at sculpturing, two hours at music, and two hours at writing each day. He broke his work into two-hour increments and his production was fantastic. Two hours at one task is usually the peak of your interest span and efficiency. If you'll put yourself on a work schedule such as this, you'll find at the end of six months, your productivity has vastly increased.

The problem is, we get under the pressure of a task and we end up spending twelve or fourteen hours a day on that job. In that situation our productivity, efficiency, and work quality drop tremendously. This principle is not only true for blue-and white-collar workers, it is especially relevant to top executives as well.

One more point, while we're on this general subject. Begin to plan your retirement at least by the time you reach fifty. If you wait until you're sixty-five, it will be most difficult for you to survive retirement—you'll fold in a heap and fade away quickly, due to the radical change in your life-style. Begin retiring in your mind, preferably fifteen years before you reach actual retirement age. Begin doing those things you are going to do when you retire. In this way, when quitting time finally comes, you'll be ready for it.

What Kind of Exercise Are You Getting?

The second part of physical fitness (after adequate rest), is exercise. What kind of physical activity are you involved in? Do you have a regular program of exercise? This is important for people who sit behind desks all day, as opposed to the man who's out digging ditches or pouring concrete. He obviously gets a good amount of physical activity.

There are two basic principles in an exercise program. First, is what we might call L-S-D (and I'm not talking about the drug). This stands for Long-Slow-Distance. You should spend approximately forty minutes to an hour, three or four times a week, in your fitness program. The goal of this exercise is stamina.

How long you exercise is much more important than how far you go. Dr. Ernst Van Aaken, who has trained more world-class athletes and marathon runners than any other living person, maintains it is the long-slow-distance that brings the best fitness results.

Fitness takes time. For the beginner, I think walking is the best exercise you can do because you can do it anywhere, at any time of the night or day. Obviously, walking doesn't have the limits that tennis or golf or swimming do.

When you begin to work at fitness your only competitor should be yourself. If you are playing tennis or handball, you are really not allowed to go at your own pace, to slow down and rest when you need to. Most of us are not interested in running a marathon or being a tennis champion. Exercise should be done for fitness' sake.

The more vigorous sports activity can be done for the sake of having a good time. Usually you cannot build vigor and stamina at the same time.

The second basic principle in your fitness program is to spend a ten-minute period in which you perform your "Interval Stress Activity" (that is, doing interval-timed stress). This is vigorous physical activity to get your heart beating at an optimum rate. Your pulse is probably the best measure of how well you are building your physical fitness. Your activity can be running, race walking, calisthenics, swimming, tennis—whatever you prefer. But it should be done with considerable vigor for ten minutes in order to get your heartbeat up and your lungs working; you will have to breathe rapidly and pant. Ten minutes of this kind of vigorous activity will do wonders for your physical fitness.

Always warm up slowly for this Interval Stress Activity. Then begin to walk fast, swinging your arms, or jog hard if you are a jogger. Push yourself, until you are breathing hard and your pulse is pounding, then slack off a bit until your heart and lungs get caught up. Repeat this cycle of push and and coast through the ten minutes or more of your I-S-A routine.

Never charge through the last 100 yards of running activity, and then collapse at your doorstep. Overdoing like that has a negative tearing-down effect on the body. The object of your Interval Stress Activity is to improve your heart and lung fitness. Your L-S-D program is to improve your overall body musculo-skeletal fitness and stamina.

Some Exercise "Dos" and "Don'ts"

There are several things I would suggest for your stamina-building exercise program. *First, don't overdo it.* One of the biggest mistakes people make in starting an exercise program is to "overdo it" at the beginning. The beginner should not charge into any fitness program as if it had to be completed yesterday. Whether you're twenty or forty or even sixty-five, start slow and build yourself up.

More people quit their fitness program because they get exhausted and have a miserable, hurting time. After each exercise period, you should feel as good or better than when you started. In my opinion, any time you end an exercise period stiff and sore and exhausted, something's wrong. Either you're sick or you're over-doing it.

One criterion you can use in your L-S-D stamina-building exer-cising is the extent of your breathing. Panting is usually too much. Ideally you should be able to breathe in through your nose and out through your mouth. You should also be able to carry on a normal conversation while you're exercising.

Second, always exercise when it's cool. I see these business execu-tives out at noon, in the heat of the day, not realizing they are ask-ing for trouble. In our local area, a football player died from heat stroke on a very hot day. If you overdo it on a hot day, you are ask-ing for trouble, even a heat stroke or a heart attack.

Third, exercise when you are hungry. Never, never exercise on a full stomach. Many of those people you read about, who have dropped dead while jogging, were running on a full stomach. Those who run in the heat of the day with a full stomach are courting all kinds of trouble. When you have food in your intestines, the body diverts up to a third of the body's total blood supply to the stomach and intestine. This deprives the skeletal muscles and heart of the maximum availability of blood with its oxygen and nutrients—the energy chemicals these organs need to work properly in a physical-exertion situation.

Fourth, don't exercise—particularly run—in the dark in unfamil-iar territory. It is too easy to sprain an ankle or break a leg by step-ping into a chuck hole.

Fifth, use footwear that fits you, and which is designed for your activity. This is especially true for runners.

Sixth, dress properly. In the summer, a heavy, tight sweat shirt and pants will heat you up and restrict cooling and evaporation. This could cause dehydration and heat stroke. In the winter, shorts and a thin shirt may cause you to chill and get sick. There is also the possibility of developing frostbite and/or hypothermia.

What About the Professional Athlete?

In my practice I have cared for a number of top athletes—among them, many of the Athletes in Action basketball, wrestling, track, and soccer players. When dealing with these athletes, we're talking about a totally different situation, because these men have built themselves into a fitness state in which they can exercise hard with little ill effects.

However, even a professional athlete can push himself to the point of utter exhaustion. Keeping at his strenous workouts day in and day out, with no breaks to give his body time to rejuvenate, can "burn out" an athlete. I remember one decathlon man who was working at his AIA ministry, as well as practicing daily. He'd been three years without a break and was at the end of his stamina. Then he caught the flu and it took three months for his body to recover.

I once had the pleasure of listening to Dr. Thomas K. Cureton, professor emeritus of physical education, at the University of Illinois, and consultant to Olympic coaches and athletes for thirty or forty years. He related how a runner, Roger Bannister, came to him for consultation, because he was struggling to break the four-minute-mile barrier. Dr. Cureton suggested he stop all heavy workouts for two to three months. He told the runner to keep himself fit but stop pushing for a while. When Bannister was renewed and the fatigue was out of his system, he was able to become the first man to run a four-minute mile.

This runner was only able to achieve this goal by letting his mind and body rest, so it could return to peak ability. You can't work out day after day, month after month, and expect good results. The rest cycle is important. The body can't do anything all the time without suffering for it.

The Weekend Athlete

Weekend athletes are quite prone to injuries. I remember one fellow who had been a good basketball player in college, but at thirty-two he had a desk job and played only on Saturdays. One weekend, as he jumped hard to shoot a basket, he came down awkwardly on his left foot. Pain went knifing through his heel; he had completely severed his Achilles tendon. This man still had the general ability he had had in college, but he didn't have the conditioning. He couldn't maintain the muscle and tendon strength he used to have on a once-a-week exercise regime.

It's the weekend baseball player, trying to outdo himself, who slides into second and breaks his leg. He doesn't have the fitness and stamina, *or* the tendon strength, to take those energy surges. For fitness, it is better to play for the "fun of it," rather than have the supercompetitive, "I've got to be number one" state of mind.

What Does It Mean to Be Fit?

The hundred-yard-dash runner uses muscle fibers that are called "fast-twitch" fibers. The marathon runner, on the other hand, uses what are called "slow-twitch" muscle fibers. The sprinter, weight lifter, and some football players have great strength and can be superactive for five to ten seconds, but most usually don't have the stamina to perform over long periods of time.

A hundred-yard-dash person may breathe once or twice in the ten seconds of the race. His heart rate at the end may get up to 150 to 160 beats a minute—only fifteen beats during the entire race! That simply isn't the stamina type of fitness.

In fitness, your first concern is your cardiovascular system. Your heart is the most essential muscle in your body. It's good to have the rest of your muscles fit, but if your heart is not fit, the rest of your body isn't worth much. No matter how good your legs and arms and back are, if you don't have a good heart, you're not fit.

This is why calisthenics by themselves are not that beneficial in building fitness. Most people who do just calisthenics are not able to work out long enough at these vigorous exercises to build stamina and cardio-pulmonary fitness. How long can you do push-ups? How long can you jump rope? How long can you do sit-ups? All of these exercises may have their place in warming you up for other activities, but they cannot stand alone for the average person. An executive, a housewife, or a businessman needs total-body fitness rather than bulging muscles or superstrength.

The Best Exercise?

The best all-around exercise, in my opinion, is walking. Stride walking or race walking is the very best. I believe that for a forty-five or fifty-year-old person to try to get out and jog is asking for trouble. The problem is they haven't used their ankles, knees, hips, and backs for many years. When they begin the steady thud-thud-thud of running on pavement, there is a great tendency to injure the legs and back. (*See* Illustration A.)

If you've ever watched stride walkers, you see them swing their arms vigorously, as they glide over the ground. You can generate as much—if not more—energy and fitness with stride walking—without anywhere near the hazard of injury of jogging, tennis, or other sports.

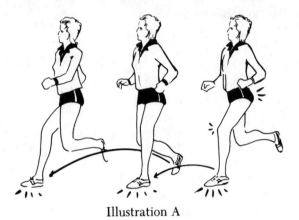

Illustration A

If you want to jog and run marathons, begin by walking, then slowly work up to a walk-jog state. If you are forty or fifty years old, do this very slowly. It should take three to six months before you are jogging a couple of miles a day. The slower you build up to it, the better off you are and the less likely you are to overdo it, injure yourself, and drop out. Again, at the end of your exercise workout, you should have a feeling of increased well-being and uplift. If your exercise makes you feel good, the chances are you will continue your exercise program.

If you decide to progress into jogging, it is essential to have running shoes that are properly fitted to support your feet and cushioned to absorb the impact. Also, find a place to run that is not concrete or asphalt. The jarring effect of hard surfaces can be quite damaging. Even hard earth next to the road is better than pavement.

Do You Know How to Breathe?

Most of us really don't know how to breathe correctly. We've developed bad habits down through the years, since infancy. We tend to hold our breath and strain. This is very unnatural and not the way we breathed when we were infants. I'm going to give you a very simple breathing exercise to do four or five times each day to increase your fitness and energy. You'll also find this exercise to be most relaxing and rejuvenating.

Stand up and let your arms and hands hang loose at your sides. Slowly raise your hands in front of you. As you do, begin to inhale. Slowly, slowly, bring your arms up, continuing to inhale. When they are all the way over your head, let them spread apart slightly until they form a V with your body. Bounce your arms backward two or three times, as far as they will go. At the same time, breathe in a little deeper with each bounce. This will lift the muscles and ribs in the upper front of your chest, allowing you to take deeper breaths.

Now let your arms drop in front of you and forcibly exhale. As you exhale, push your abdominal muscles back against your backbone and up under your rib cage with a forcible, expiratory, audible *swoosh*. (*See* Illustration *B*.) Don't allow your shoulders and chest to drop forward in a slump position as you exhale. The forward bend in your torso should come in the lower part of your chest and the upper part of your abdomen and your lower back. Tuck your buttocks in under you and push your stomach muscles in and up and back, rather than just bending forward.

In this way, you use three of the basic areas of breathing: (1) the lower abdominal; (2) the upper abdomen, lower sides of the chest;

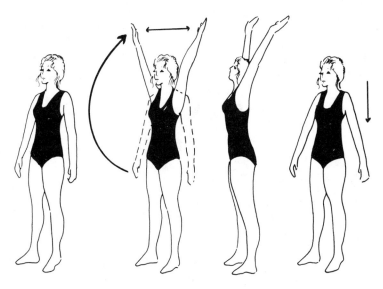

Illustration B

and (3) the upper front of your chest. Do this exercise two or three times, and you will notice you will dramatically improve the circulation all over your body, particularly to your brain. This is a very relaxing tension-relieving exercise.

A General Body Toner

Several years ago I found an exercise that tones the body, particularly the abdominal wall. It is a Chinese isometric exercise. Stand with your feet parallel and comfortably twelve to eighteen inches apart, depending on your build. Your toes should be straight or even pointing slightly inward.

Bend your knees slightly, so your leg and thigh and buttock muscles are carrying your weight. Tuck your pelvis in under your body. Tighten, push in and upward with your abdominal muscles. Hold your chest and head up. Push your chin gently backwards, then push your shoulders out laterally. Hold your elbows out three to four inches from your body and slightly forward. Bend your elbows, so your cupped hands are face up and about belt-high.

Now tense all the muscles in your body, particularly your tummy muscles. Hold this stance for as long as you can. Repeat it two or

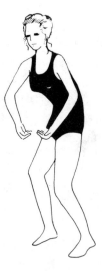

Illustration C

three times. While doing the exercise, only take shallow, small breaths. (*See* Illustration *C*.)

Shoulder-Back Stretches

Stand with your feet moderately apart. Grasp a rope or towel and raise your arms over your head, so they form a rather wide V. (*See* Illustration *D*.) Holding your elbows stiff, pull first to the right then to the left. Swing your arms back and forth while they are behind your head and shoulders. Keep your elbows stiff. Pull on the upright arm, so the arm and shoulder stretch across, over, and somewhat behind the head. Do this four or five times.

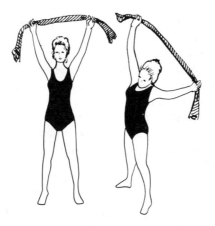

Illustration D

A variation of this exercise is the see-saw. Using the same stance and rope or towel, start with V position, but this time, pull with one arm and bend the other at the elbow, using a steady tension. See-saw back and forth bringing the rope or towel down across the back, until your arms are down to your sides. (*See* Illustration *E*.)

What About Dehydration and Salt Tablets?

It is a good idea, before you go out for your exercise period to hydrate yourself somewhat by drinking juice, tea, or water. This

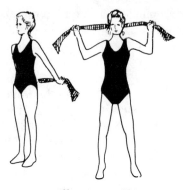

Illustration E

will help you stay ahead of the dehydration process that comes from sweating while exercising. Water in your stomach is not going to divert the blood supply from the heart.

A common problem I find in professional athletes, particularly in wrestlers, is their need to constantly meet their weight limitations. They will stop eating and drinking, and go to the furnace room, where they can sweat off four or five pounds in order to meet their weight requirement. This can have a very detrimental effect on the body. Not eating and drinking coupled with heavy sweating may cause a severe loss of the mineral potassium. Low potassium levels in the blood cause extreme weakness and nausea, even heart irregularities. If you exercise often and sweat a lot, you may want to take a potassium supplement to make certain you are not depleted in this needed element. You should also know that taking too much potassium can be harmful to your heart and muscles.

Hydrating yourself *before* you begin your workout is a good idea. If you are going to exercise early in the morning, when you first get up, I believe a warm liquid, like hot tea or warm juice, is much better than something ice-cold. Warmth soothes and relaxes. It doesn't shock the body. It also promotes circulation, while cold chills and causes constriction of the blood vessels. Putting two glasses of ice-cold liquid into your stomach early in the morning has a very negative effect on the body. Drinking something cold on a hot afternoon is a different story, but early in the morning, try to avoid cold drinks.

How much should you drink after you've exercised? Of course, this depends on how much and how long you exercised and your state of dehydration before you began. For you to have an eight-ounce glass or two to drink at the end of an activity period is usually sufficient. But if you were to drink six or eight eight-ounce glasses all at one time, you might hyperhydrate yourself. This would tend to have a toxic negative effect on your system. Let your body be your guide. Drink some, then wait. If you're still thirsty, drink more.

What About Injuries?

The first thing you should do when you pull a muscle or sprain an ankle, is to ice it. Never use heat on a fresh injury. It is also most important in the initial stages of an injury to rest the injured part. If you have injured a leg, try not to walk on it. A 150-pound body walking on a sprained ankle exerts a tremendous amount of pressure. You should wait until you can move the part easily, and bear weight or pressure without significant discomfort before beginning to use it again.

The criterion I use with professional athletes for the first ten to fourteen days is, if it hurts a lot after you use it—you are pushing too fast. You are probably creating more injury.

If you have swelling, elevate the injured part. In the first forty-eight hours, make certain you use only nonstress motion. Supporting the part with an ace bandage in the acute stage is important, so that you don't overly stress it. At this point you can often begin hot-then-cold soaks. Heat the injury for four or five minutes, then soak it in cold water for two or three. Repeat this several times. This has a pumping action. Heat helps bring in good, fresh blood, and cold pumps out the old congestion and swelling.

A common misconception I hear from people is, "Well I can move it, so I guess it's not broken." Don't believe it. I have had a number of patients come into my office walking on a broken ankle. Of course, see your physician if there is any doubt about the injury. He will probably want to X-ray it to make certain it isn't broken.

Your Posture

While we're discussing physical fitness, how's your posture? I believe the key idea in posture is to "sit tall" and "stand tall." Perhaps you are old enough to remember the cartoons of GI Joe in World War II. His chin was high. His chest was thrust out front and his shoulders were back. He had a big curve in his lower back. Actually, that is a miserable posture.

Posture begins in your feet. It is difficult to have good posture, if you wear shoes with heels that are too high. High heels tend to throw the rest of the body into a forward imbalance. They create many leg, knee, and low-back problems for women. Short women, who vainly try to be tall by wearing very high heels, often suffer from foot and low-back problems. The high heels tend to jam the toes into the front of the shoe. They also tend to cause sway-back and chronic low-back pain.

Some bad postures are caused by flat feet. If one foot is flatter than the other, it tends to shorten one leg. If you have flat feet, you should wear shoes that give good support, especially in the arches.

Very often the person who stands with one shoulder higher than the other, with his head bent to one side and his body twisted a little, is doing so because of a structural problem. It's not just because they've developed a bad habit. A person who has one leg that's an inch shorter than the other has a natural tendency to stand with his back curved in a scoliosis.

To ascertain "what's not right" about your posture, stand unclothed in front of a mirror and look at yourself. Imagine there is a vertical line that drops from the ceiling right in front of your nose to the floor. Is one shoulder higher than the other? Is one ear lower? Can you see a curvature in your body? Do you stand with one shoulder forward? Do you seem to slump on one side more than the other? These are all structural problems. If you have chronic musculoskeletal problems, find yourself a good osteopath or chiropractor who uses the sacro-occipital technique of Dr. Bertrand DeJarnette, of Nebraska City, Nebraska.

Another important factor in good posture is your eyes. They are always oriented to be horizontal to the horizon. If you had one shoe on and one off, you would automatically bend your head, neck, and back so your eyes were horizontal to the horizon. A person with a posture imbalance tends to adjust his stance, so he can look evenly at the horizon.

The next area most likely to cause posture problems is your low

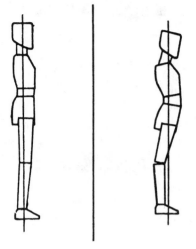

Illustration F

back and pelvis. The forward tilt of the pelvis increases the front-to-back curve in the lower spine. This is what is called a sway-back. (*See* Illustration *F*.) It is usually just a lazy posture, though it can be a true structural problem. This problem is created by standing in a relaxed position, letting the abdominal muscles slump, making a potbelly. This allows the low back to sway forward sloppily. This is not the way we were designed, and it puts an undue strain on the back. Many such problems are simply due to poor muscle tone in the abdomen and buttock muscles. A big belly is often due as much to flabby muscle as it is to fat.

The first thing to do to correct this pelvic posture problem is to stand about two feet back from a desk or table (more, if you are a tall person). Bend at your hips and place your hands on the top of a chair. To start, you exaggerate the problem and increase the curvature in your low back. (That is, increase the low-back sway or curve. Overdoing the problem helps you understand what's wrong.) Then tighten your buttock muscles. Make believe you are holding a hundred-dollar bill in the crease between your buttocks, and that you must hold on to it tightly or lose it. Then tighten your abdominal muscles and tip your pelvis up in front and move it forward

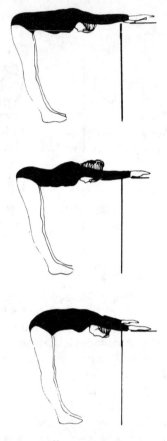

Illustration G

under your torso. This brings your pelvis in underneath your spine
in such a way that you can stand with it being balanced. (*See* Illustrations in **G.**)

When you stand, you should stand with your chest up, your pelvis tipped up in front, and your chin up and back. Your tummy
muscles should be tucked up and in, and you should balance easily
on the balls of your feet rather than on your heels. Put as much
weight on your toes and the balls of your feet as you do on your
heels. Be sure you can feel all five of your toes pressing against the
floor—they should be pointed just slightly inward.

The Hula

A good exercise to improve your posture and help you loosen your pelvic muscles, ligaments, and joints is the hula. Stand with your feet ten to twelve inches apart. Your head and feet should stay relatively in the same place. Move your pelvis to one side, so your body bends in the middle forming a V. Move your pelvis in as wide a circle as you can: side-front-side-back. Remember, try to keep your head as close to a midline point over your feet as you can. (*See* Illustration *H.*) This is not an exercise in which you rotate your head and torso around your pelvis. That exercise can be very aggravating to low-back problems. (A good book for those of you with low-back problems is *Dr. Thompson's New Way for You to Cure Your Aching Back*, by Jess Stearn (Doubleday & Co., Inc.)

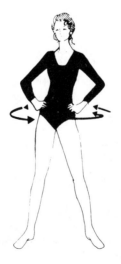

Illustration H

III
Dealing With the
Emotional Problems

10
What Are Your Deepest Hurts?

"Into each life some rain must fall." Everyone experiences deep hurts. Our deepest hurts most often come from those that are closest to us. If we love someone, we're bound to be hurt by them. Each of us has had deep disappointments and traumatic experiences. If we've been physically attacked, we may respond with terror at the slightest threat of physical harm. The unresolved deep hurts in your past affect you today. They color everything you feel and do. It is important for you to become aware of what these hurts are so you can release them.

In the past month, I have asked two of my clinical psychiatrist friends if they could remember a deep hurt or a big disappointment they suffered in the past. Both of them responded almost instantly, giving details of a hurt that happened twenty or thirty years before. When one of the doctors finished his story, he said, "That's funny. I haven't thought of that incident for years and years."

You would think a psychiatrist, who had been practicing fifteen years, would have his hurts pretty well resolved. Not so. Nor is it true for most of the rest of the world either. I've only had one patient who couldn't remember any deep hurt or big disappointment.

Many times my patients ask, "Why go back and dig up all that garbage in the past?" But these experiences, unless they're resolved and healed, taint our thinking and affect us today. It is better to dig up and release past hurts. No matter how unpleasant and difficult they may have been, they must be released and healed. Confession is the answer not suppression.

The First Trauma of Life

Certainly you cannot consciously remember it, but your first major traumatic experience was being born. You were quite comfortable in your mother's womb, before being thrust into the harsh light of the delivery room. You came from a totally satisfying environment into a world that's full of problems. That day was the beginning of your hurts; you probably haven't stopped kicking against the inequalities, dissatisfactions, betrayals and imperfections found in all human beings since then.

Recently there has been a new emphasis on an age-old manner of delivering a baby. A French doctor has dulled the delivery-room lights, introduced soft music, and allowed the father to be present. The child is immediately placed on its mother's tummy, where it can feel her warmth and the gentle rhythm of her breathing. Pediatricians and parents find there is a significant positive difference in children who start life with this method of delivery.

As we begin life, we are the center of our own little universe. Every thing and every one revolve around us. In a sense, we control that universe with our wants and needs, even though they are relatively simple. We need to be fed, to be touched and held, to be loved and accepted. If these needs are adequately supplied, we live. If they aren't, we die. In our earliest years of life, even the lack of being loved enough can be fatal to us.

Life is less than perfect. It's humanly impossible to receive total fulfillment of all our needs. If our needs are over or undersupplied, hurts begin to build up within us. It may be the hurt of hunger, or the hurt of not being held and touched enough. It may be the hurt of being criticized, judged unjustly, and misunderstood.

So our hurts begin at a very early age. We soon learn that those around us have inadequacies and weaknesses of their own. They are less than the "perfect creatures" we fantasize them to be. Many of our parents' hungers and hurts have not been resolved or healed. They didn't learn how to love, because they weren't loved enough by their parents; they are therefore unable to completely meet and satisfy the needs in our lives.

Unsatisfied needs that linger on as hurts and disappointments tend to cause us to doubt, disbelieve, and be fearful. Unresolved gaps in our emotional makeup cloud our thinking. What you are now is the product of what you thought yesterday, a year ago, ten years ago. How you see yourself is the result of how you have been programmed and conditioned. Our tendency to see ourselves in a negative light is learned through our life experiences which have left us feeling wanting, empty, inferior, and of poor self-worth.

Pain From the Past

Most of our lingering hurts come from emotional blows over which we had no control. There was a woman in my office recently who was bound by a horribly negative self-image. She had been to several psychiatrists for treatment but had not received much help. As we were talking, I asked, "What is a big hurt in your life?"

Immediately she became quiet. Tears came to her eyes and she said slowly, "Well . . . I was conceived out of wedlock. My mother and father got married because of me. Mother used to yell at me, 'If it hadn't been for you, I wouldn't be in this mess.' When I was twelve, both my parents abandoned me and left me with relatives."

Talk about pain. A sense of rejection saturated this woman's self-image. It so affected her chemistry that she had many physical problems. Her greatest need was for a very painful memory to be healed. Memories are chemistry. Bad feelings cause bad chemistry—and bad chemistry makes us hurt all over.

Another recent patient told me of her extremely abnormal cravings for sugar. "I think I would kill for a candy bar," she said quite matter-of-factly.

When this woman got into one of her sugar-craving moods, she would get up in the middle of the night and raid the cupboards for anything sweet; she would often eat a whole pound of brown sugar. If there was nothing sweet in the house, she would go to the corner market and buy ten candy bars and devour them all before going back to bed. She had an absolutely uncontrolled craving for sugar.

When we began to talk about the deep hurts in this lady's life, she revealed that from the time she was six until she was eleven, her father and another man in the household had used her sexually. When a child, especially at such a young, formative age, is betrayed and exploited for sexual purposes by her own father, a tremendous emotional hurt results. Those hurts can only be resolved through an emotional-spiritual healing. (This woman's situation was certainly not an exception. Most sexual molestation is done by close members of the family.)

Basically, this lady was seeking love. She gained a pseudo-satisfaction through the gratification of eating sweets, but it didn't satisfy her deep sense of bitterness, anger, hatred and betrayal toward her father.

One of the things I try to explain in this kind of situation is that a father who would sexually abuse a young child has to be emotionally, mentally, spiritually, and physically sick. A person truly in their right mind would never do something like that.

Another patient responded to my question about a hurt in her past, "Yes, I can remember something. I don't clearly remember what it was all about. It happened when I was three and a half."

She didn't elaborate, so I said, "Can you tell me more?"

"Yes. It happened out in the backyard."

"Is this something that involved you sexually?"

"Yes . . . yes it was."

"Did it hurt?"

"Oh, yes, it *really* hurt, now that I think about it." Then she added, "You know, I haven't thought about that in years." The incident happened fifty years ago, and she claimed she had forgotten about it. But it's my impression this deep hurt was still affecting her with some very negative chemistry. Such "hurts" stay in our subconscious and are always waiting to spring to the surface, until they are released and healed.

A fact that constantly amazes me is the speed with which people remember the hurts they have suffered. I remember another woman whom I asked about her past experiences. Within seconds she replied, "Well yes, I remember when I was four years of age, I was kidnapped. I haven't thought of that for years. I can still feel the terror I experienced, as I was being driven away in that horse and buggy. But Dad jumped on his horse and caught up and rescued me."

This was a fearful, apprehensive woman. I don't know how much of her current problems found their roots in that childhood experience, but I'm sure some did.

Another patient revealed to me her father had died when she was five. She was still hurting over this loss, which had never been resolved. She feared others would not love her, and was still actually feeling rejected by her father. The fact that he had no control over his death didn't really matter to her. The empty void of not having a father was still there.

There's more to the healing of our bad-memory chemistry than just coming to accept these hurts and learning to live with them. There cannot be wholeness in the body, until there is healing and forgiveness from the heart. It is important to realize we must accept and release the emotional hurts of our past if we are to have a healthy future.

Take a New Look at Your Parents

Many, many of our early problems can be traced back to our parents. Because they did not have all their needs met, they were not able to meet all of ours. To be able to deal adequately with the past, we must be able to take a new and honest look at our parents.

Most of us have a deep sense of loyalty to our parents. As small children, we see them as omnipotent and able to do anything. As we grow older, their imperfections become apparent. Their halos tarnish and chip; they become people with inadequacies and weaknesses who fail us.

Parents often tend to try to perpetuate this godlike image by saying: "I'm your father, mind me!" "Don't question what I tell you to do." When something goes wrong, they may explain it wasn't their fault.

It is very difficult to release our fantasies of perfection and learn to be realistic about mother and father. We want them to be perfect—but they are not perfect. We want them to be all-powerful—but they are not all-powerful. Eventually we must be honest with ourselves and face the fact our parents are human.

God wants you to love, honor, cherish, and obey your parents. He wants you to be loyal to them—but you do not need to love or be loyal to everything they do. In fact, you can and should dislike some of their ways. You need to accept them as frail, finite human beings—not little gods.

One of the best definitions of love I know came from a child. He said, "Love is when someone knows the worst about you but loves you just the same." Be willing to face the worst in your parents; be willing to see their faults. Then love them for what they are, not for what they do. Try to see and feel the deep hurts in their lives. Isn't that how God loves us?

How's Your Self-Image?

A few years ago, a plastic surgeon named Maxwell Maltz found that people's personalities often changed dramatically when their facial appearances were improved by surgery. Dr. Maltz realized that these people now saw themselves as "attractive" and began to behave with a greater sense of confidence toward themselves.

But not everyone he changed surgically changed emotionally. Many patients continued to see themselves as "unattractive," and acted accordingly. Dr. Maltz realized that how a person feels about himself is far more important to his well-being than actually how attractive or unattractive his appearance is to others.

What a person does "for fun" can be a good indicator of his self-image. I like to ask my patients, "What do you do for fun? Are you a happy person?" The answers to these questions go a long way toward revealing a person's sense of self-worth and wholeness. If you have a positive self-concept, and a positive self-expectancy, then you have good chemistry. If you have a negative self-image, then you have bad chemistry going on within your body—there is tension and conflict present, and that's self-destructive.

Your self-image is every bit as important to your health as whether or not you have blood in your stools or headaches. How you see yourself is extremely important to your emotional well-being.

I remember hearing of a young boy who had been admitted to a mental institution. He became tremendously depressed and began to behave in a bizarre manner. He was classified as "severely disturbed." A Christian, who was not a psychiatrist, went to see the boy and discovered the boy's major problem was simply that he thought he was "ugly," because two other boys had told him so.

Once the boy realized he was normal, his severe emotional disturbance began to resolve itself.

When I sense a patient has a negative self-image, I ask, "Why do
you care so little about yourself?" "Why are you so down on yourself?"

The answers I receive often sound like this: "I was never allowed
to have fun as a child. To have fun was to be sinful. We always had
to work." Most of this type of thinking relates back to early childhood training and experiences. Often the person was verbally and
nonverbally put down as a child; or he picked up the nonverbal attitudes of the parents, looking down on anything that was fun.

I was counseling with a young man who was having a difficult
time adjusting to his young marriage and life in general. Most of his
problems related back to the fact that he had received much disap-
proval from his parents. With tears in his eyes, he told me,
"Straight *A*'s weren't good enough!" His parents had such perfec-
tionist and negative attitudes that there wasn't anything he could
do to earn their acceptance and approval. As a result, he had never
felt the assurance of his own self-worth. Consequently, he had tremendous feelings of inferiority.

In this area of self-image, problems are centered in trying to be
something we are not. We have a need to be pleasing to other people. In failing to feel we are acceptable to others, we experience
rejection and unhappiness. When we don't live up to the expectations of others, we can become deeply hurt by their nonacceptance.

Hatred is really hating hatred. Hostility is hostility toward hostility. Anger is being angry over anger in ourselves as well as in other
people. Resentment is resenting resentment. All of these emotions
come when we are hurt and rejected. They seem to feed back and
nourish themselves, each breeding more of what it is. When a seed
of bitterness starts within us, unless we resolve that hurt, it tends to
grow and becomes a mind-obsessing, self-perpetuating problem.
You become what your thoughts focus on. What you feed your
mind, or what you allow others to feed it, is what you are. Our actions are the result of our attitudes.

Ultimately, happiness and having fun is a state of mind. If I like
myself and like what I'm doing, then that's what counts most.
Being happy and having fun are high on my priority list, because I
know they are an essential part of good health.

Where Do We Go for Love?

Supporting and maintaining physical life is a constant "do-it-yourself" activity. No one is going to breathe for you, or eat for you, or walk for you, or talk for you. You have to do it all yourself.

The paradox is that, in the emotional side of life, being loved is not something we can do for ourselves. It is something we must do for other people, and which they must do for us. The fact that you have lived to be a teenager or an adult means you have experienced love. You have to experience it before you can give it.

But if you have deep unfulfilled needs for love because you have not been loved adequately in the past, you will tend to focus on the empty side of your life. You will seek to get love by various manipulations of others. Not being loved enough is painful, and we tend to focus on that hurt. We hunger for love, but the more we seek it, the more we repel it.

In my opinion, all our emotional hurts can be traced back to a lack of love. We all have a feeling of not being loved enough, to a greater or lesser degree. This is only natural, because no human being can love someone "enough." There is always a deficiency. Failure to love enough is the common denominator in all human beings. *Failing to love is sin.*

Man's deepest need is to be loved enough, to be accepted, approved, and forgiven unconditionally. This is also man's biggest disappointment and deepest hurt. "Humanly speaking," these are impossible obstacles to overcome. But, with God, all things are possible, for the power of God is His love.

11
The Bad Chemistry of Negative Feelings

Feelings Affect Your Whole Body

All emotions are expressed one way or another through our physical body. Bad feelings produce bad chemistry and sooner or later, these feelings manifest themselves in physical problems. The bad chemistry of anger, bitterness, and hatred tend to create negative tension and dis—ease. These emotions raise blood pressure and cause circulatory disturbances, ulcers, colitis, skin rashes, headaches, heart attacks, and a host of other dis—eases. The constant effect of this negative chemistry also depletes the adrenal glands— the shock absorbers of the body.

On the positive side, feelings of self-confidence, joy, happiness, and peace of mind, all tend to create a sense of ease within the body. These emotions allow the body to function at optimum capacity without any restriction. These good chemistry feelings tend to help our neurological and endocrine systems to function at their optimum levels. When you are happy and relaxed, you are free of negative muscular tension. When you are at peace with yourself, you can play and work in a much more efficient manner than a person who is compulsively uptight.

Many top athletes can tell you of a time when they played their best, without having to think or worry about their game. Their actions and reactions were almost automatic. They may have been trying to put out only about 80 percent of their ability, but because they were relaxed and confident, they performed at their highest level of ability.

The opposite is true on the day when the athlete is upset or in a bad mood. Perhaps he is trying too hard and has an intense preoccupation with what he is doing and how to act and react. Consequently, he makes more mistakes than normally. This type of problem is certainly not limited to athletes.

You would probably be amazed at the number of patients who come into my office who have developed physical problems based on their bad feelings toward others. Whether it is an ulcer, insomnia, or high blood pressure, sooner or later this bad chemistry of negative feelings begins to produce physical symptoms and dis—ease.

God knows this and He says, "Anxiety in the heart of a man weighs it down . . ." (Proverbs 12:25). He also tells us it is harder for a man to bear up under emotional pain than it is to endure sickness (Proverbs 18:14). If your mind is preoccupied with hurts, on the injustices that have happened to you, you will eventually have physical dis—ease.

I recall one woman who had a serious stomach problem, nervous tension, and sleeplessness. Her husband had left her for another woman, and she was having a difficult time adjusting to the emotional upheaval it had brought. She told me, "It makes me so mad! They're out there having a good time, and I'm hurting!"

She was hurting because of the hatred she felt towards her former husband and the other woman. His betrayal and rejection had caused her to have a very negative sense of self-worth. She was having many physical problems because she had accepted the negative image he had imposed on her, by his rejection.

Have You Developed Negative Thought Patterns?

Doubt, denial, and disbelief cloud your mental picture of yourself and confuse your thinking about life. Even the slightest element of disbelief tends to make you a doubting, negative-minded person.

An idea that becomes fixed in the mind, one which you think about all the time, will eventually come true. If you have a fear which is constantly on your mind, there is a tendency for that fear to come to pass. If you are afraid you are not going to be loved, you will probably erect subtle barriers in your personality that will drive away the very love you desire.

You may fearfully visualize something bad happening. "I just know I'm going to have an accident," "I'll never find a parking place," or "I just know I'm going to get sick." The more you visualize that fear, and the more you believe it, the more likely it is to happen.

You've heard of accident-prone people. It's true. A small percentage of people are involved in the majority of all accidents. The same is true with sickness. Less than 25 percent of the population accounts for more than 75 percent of all doctors' visits. People who "think well" tend to stay well. People who "think sick" tend to get sick more often.

I had a woman in my office who had unresolved hurts stemming from her early childhood. They were major causative factors in her current medical problems. Her mother had often overtly stated that her happiness or unhappiness depended upon what she, as a little girl, did or didn't do. Now, in adult life, she still felt responsible for the happiness of her husband and family; if they weren't happy, she felt it was because she hadn't done the right things. Of course, this is quite unrealistic, for no one can *make* someone else happy.

This woman's mind had been programmed with fear that she would not be able to make her loved ones happy. Consequently her self-doubting, fearful attitude caused so much tension that there was constant conflict in her home—and nobody was happy.

An opening comment of another woman, an attractive, immaculately dressed mother of five, came to me as a complete surprise. "I believe I should tell you I'm a controlled alcoholic," she said. "I went into modeling to please my father. Because drinking was a part of my occupation, I soon became an alcoholic, just like my father, even though I despised this weakness in him."

Many patients tell me how they hate or despise an attitude or negative behavioral trait in a loved one. "I'm never going to be that way," they emphatically explain. But because of this obsessive negative focus, that is exactly what they end up doing.

I was counseling, recently, with a twenty-eight-year-old man with a serious type of arthritis and blood-pressure condition. His whole countenance and body carriage exuded stress and anxiety. There was little in his life he wasn't worried about. As I talked with him, he shared that his life was all work and no play. Several times he rather vehemently stated, "I'm not going to be like my father!"

I pointed out to him that his fear of being like his father was enslaving him. His constant striving *not* to do things "like Dad" was predisposing him to be what he didn't want to be. It was also creating a negative tension and adverse chemistry in him which were a significant part of his physical ailments.

A couple of months later, when he was much improved, he remarked, "I think what helped me the most was your helping me to see my very negative attitude toward myself and life in general. Just "letting go" has made a big difference."

Fear of the Future

Many of our emotional problems come out of our apprehension of the future. We tend to fear the unknown. One of the most universal fears is the fear of death. Very few people ever completely resolve this fear. It can subtly dominate our thinking, in one way or the other. In some people, this fear becomes so overwhelming and debilitating, the person becomes a total recluse. Because of their fear of death, they blank out most of the rest of life. This problem will never be resolved in our thinking until it is faced in complete self-honesty. It will dominate your life, creating negative chemistry, until it is resolved.

Ernest Becker in his book *Escape From Evil* proposes with sound evidence, that man's deepest motivation is the fear of death. The greatest evil is to try to avoid death by promoting one's own life at the expense of others.

Much of what we do is motivated by our fear of death. We obey traffic signs and signals, because we know if we don't there is a possibility we may be killed in an auto accident. We go to work, not so much because we enjoy working, as because we are afraid we won't have enough money to buy food and to keep a roof over our heads.

But death isn't the only thing we fear in the future; we often fear just change itself. We may worry over how the years will affect our looks, our earning power, or our ability to cope. Alvin Toffler introduced the concept of "future shock" in his best-selling book of the same name. Future shock is really a crisis in self-esteem. We worry, "Will I be able to handle that change when it comes?" In essence, our self-worth is being assaulted. As we fret and worry about the problem, bad chemistry is created in our bodies.

We see the actions of terrorist groups, civil strife, and international kidnappings documented on our television screens within a few hours of their actual happening. Our newspapers and magazines are filled with murders, rapes, airplane crashes, and the mass-induced suicides by the Jim Jones cult. And if the newscasts aren't enough, we have highly dramatized versions depicted on many "entertainment" programs.

It's been said we live in the Age of Anxiety. Many say our century is more anxiety ridden than any other era since the Middle Ages. Anxiety is characterized by feelings of overconcern, worry, apprehension, dread, and uneasiness. The chemistry of these feelings is negative and self-destructive. If intense enough, they will lead to overt physical problems.

If you dread the future and are always apprehensive about what's around the next corner, you are living an unhappy, unsettled, and unfulfilled life. God does not want us to live in fear. "For God hath not given us the spirit of fear; but of power, and of love, and of a sound mind" (2 Timothy 1:7 KJV). He wants us to be able to face the future—and the eventuality of death—with confidence and faith.

Unexpected Emotional Problems

Many of our emotional irritations come neither out of the past nor the future. They attack us in the present—when we least expect it. None of us *plans on problems;* we live as if they are never going to come our way. But when they do, how we react is of extreme importance.

I'm convinced God is more interested in our response to life's stress situations than He is in the problems themselves. He sees problems as stepping-stones for building our character. We often see problems as fearful, unbearable obstacles to happiness and peace of mind.

What do you think of when you see someone who is angry? You think of glaring eyes, a red face, tightened fists, tension, and stress. All of that is chemistry. Have you ever changed lanes on the freeway, only to discover that the person behind you did not want you to move into "his space"? He blasts on his horn, stomps on his accelerator, and passes you in a huff, leaving you wondering why he flew into such a rage.

The apostle Paul said, "Be angry, and yet do not sin; do not let the sun go down on your anger" (Ephesians 4:26). Anger is an emotion. Emotions are not, in and of themselves, sinful. We cannot always control all of our reactions to a problem, but we certainly do not have to let an irritation grow into a major sin on our part. And we can also learn, with God's help, not to react adversely to life's situations.

Being Able to Express Emotions

As children, we are often not allowed to express our hostilities, the hurts, and disappointments, particularly those that came from parents or others in authority over us. If your parents were insecure, they had so many hurts in their lives that they were not able to allow you to respond in an angry or hostile way. Thus, you did not learn to deal with the anger, the bitterness, and the disappointments that developed deep within you.

We should be able to express and work out these hurt feelings and experiences. It is as we are able to let go of them that love can flow into our hearts in such a way that enables us to become whole people. It is important for parents to allow children to be hurt and angry, and to express their negative feelings. A child should be able to express these feelings, without having them suppressed as being bad and wrong.

The biggest argument I had with my daughter, Mona, was when she wanted to see the movie *Bonnie and Clyde*. She was twelve years old at the time and I figured that kind of blood and sex wouldn't do her mind any good. We really had a royal battle. After a long discussion, I simply said no.

She responded by saying, "Oh, you and your Jesus Christ. I hate you! I hate you! You're the most awful father in the whole world!" And she ran screaming off to her bedroom and slammed the door.

I didn't fight back or exercise my authority to demand an apology. I knew she was expressing true frustration, because I was denying her something she thought she was entitled to do. Her anger was something she had to express and get out of her system. Later, she resolved the problem in her mind and accepted my decision. In the intervening years, she has expressed to my wife and me many times how grateful she is to us for loving her enough to say no and stick by our honest convictions.

Anger is a true feeling response. But when it comes out of a deep,

deep sense of hurt, the answer isn't to club it over the head with a lot of self-criticism and then suppress it into our subconscious. Try not to let the sun go down upon your wrath. Get it out and let it go.

Remember, a parent can suppress the emotions of his children. He can force them to brood silently and angrily inside. Anger that is suppressed is transformed into depression, then bitterness, hostility, and so on. It is a major cause of youthful rebellion. It could even cause you to lose your children.

The ultimate in expressing anger is expressing your anger toward God. He is the Source and Controller of the world. To the human mind, He is the logical Person for us to become upset with, when things don't go right. In a meeting I attended some years ago, Elisabeth Elliot discussed how she had to come to grips with this conflict in herself. Deep within, she had unexpressed anger toward God. It was only when she was able to bring this up to her conscious awareness that she was able to talk about it to God. Then she was able to resolve this negative feeling.

It is so easy, either in our pride or fear, to keep such thoughts deeply hidden. Our pride tells us that others would look down on us for having such feelings. And, of course, we fear what God might do with us, if we voiced such disloyalty to Him. Perhaps we are afraid He would stop loving us and inflict more hurts on us. Of course God knows what's in our hearts, even if we don't express it. It isn't for *His* benefit that we tell Him how we feel; it's for our good. Confession is the answer, not suppression. In confession we find forgiveness and cleansing.

Learn to Deal With Your Emotions

There is no logic or reason to "feelings." Emotions cannot be logically rationalized. When we say "I hate you because . . ." our statement of cause is irrelevant. Feelings have no "becauses." They just are. It's a mentally dishonest gymnastic we go through to justify our prejudices and biases. Ultimately we are only trying to deny the human weaknesses and inadequacies within ourselves. That causes us to get angry and hate and resent and be hostile. It's a reaction to our sense of having been wronged or sinned against.

I believe we can divide all emotional responses into positive and negative chemistry. Ultimately, all negative chemistry begins first in doubt and denial, then in disobedience. There is a carnal nature within each of us—a "little god," the self-god or ego—that chooses not to believe and to disobey. Out of disobedience comes guilt. Out of guilt comes fear. Out of fear comes bitterness, anger, resentment, hatred, and hostility. All these feelings produce negative chemistry.

When Adam and Eve disobeyed and ate the fruit, they became little "self-gods" who thought they could know good from evil. Since "the Fall," this self-centered little god-man within us tends to judge every thing that hurts—or is a struggle, or denies us pleasure—as being wrong or bad. Our mind reasons, *I've been sinned against; it's unjust! It isn't right!*

If you were beaten up in a robbery, you would be hurting. But the person who was unkind and unloving to you really violated the second greatest commandment: to love his neighbor as he loves himself. His sin is failing to obey God (that is, not being loving to his neighbor). But when people are unloving, unkind, and uncompassionate towards us, our human nature immediately says, "I've been wronged!" Then we start to justify our hurt, anger, and our wish for judgment and revenge. This negative-judging reaction is the basis for causing many of the bad chemistry dis—eases in our bodies.

Our brain is like a computer. It functions by logic and reason—without feelings. The heart or emotional side of our being is solely feelings. The sense of being loved, wanted, and needed doesn't have any explanation. Likewise, the senses of rejection, bitterness, and hatred are feeling responses that don't have any logical or reasonable explanation either. Life experiences which you respond to negatively may be things which other people tend to respond to positively. It's not what happens to us that counts as much as how we react to what happens to us.

Learn to Face Your Weaknesses

We tend to have only one dominant conscious feeling at a time. When we feel angry, we feel angry all over. If we are bitter, we are bitter all over. If we're happy, we're happy all over. Negative emotions tend to dominate positive ones. It's difficult, if not impossible, to be mad and happy at the same time. So when we are rejected in one small area by someone, that rejection gives us a sense of being totally rejected. Our relationships with others at any moment are either good or bad, acceptable or unacceptable, loved or unloved.

As stated earlier in this chapter, doubt and fear tend to destroy faith and trust. Even a ½ of 1 percent doubt, can negatively influence a 99½ percent of trust. If I have even the smallest doubt you are going to fail me, then I live in fear, and sooner or later my foreboding will come true.

This is easy to overcome, however, because when I accept the fact that you are a human being, I also accept the fact that *you will fail me.* In your human weakness and inadequacy, you are not going to live up to my expectations; in fact, I have faith you will disappoint me so when it happens, I should not be surprised and disappointed. Proverbs says, "Faithful are the wounds of a friend, but deceitful are the kisses of an enemy" (27:6).

We must learn to face the reality of our negative emotions. For there to be a balance, we must have both negative and positive emotions. There is no love without hate. There is no peace without the existence of conflict. No up, without down.

The human inclination within each of us is to want to see ourselves as perfect and ideal. We'd rather just blank out and deny having any negative qualities. We tend to envision ourselves as successful in business, good husbands, good wives, good fathers and mothers. We tend to look at ourselves almost completely in the positive sense. This is very one-sided and unrealistic.

In fact, it is the weakness side of our lives that has the greatest impact on others. If I were to tell you of all of my successes, you would feel inferior. If you tell me about all your success, then I would feel inferior. However, when I share with you my weaknesses and inadequacies, and you with me, then we care and share on a horizontal level.

Each of us can identify with the weaknesses in others. As I look back in my life, the events that have had the most meaning to me are the experiences in which I made the biggest mistakes—those times when I was most certain I was right, and I actually was wrong. When I share these not-so-successful and not-so-happy experiences with others, they can identify because they've been there too.

For the past four years I have participated in a "small-group meeting" with six Christian businessmen. We meet together once a week for an hour and a half. The core of this meeting is Scripture reading, prayer, and sharing of our needs, hurts, and frustrations. In this small group, pride seems to be the biggest barrier to the sharing-healing process. My sense of logic tells me, if I share my failures with my friends, they are going to see how inadequate, weak, and worthless I am. They will look down on me; they may even reject me. Actually, the opposite is true. But it still takes far greater courage to risk being vulnerable and share your hurts, failures, and inadequacies than it does to share your successes. Being honest about oneself builds respect. It is something other people relate to and admire. In the long run, we have a greater sense of acceptance among ourselves, because we have been willing to be open and share, out of our deep hurts.

Let God Make Up the Difference

If when I get angry, I blame my anger on one of my children or my wife, I'm being very dishonest. No matter what they did to irritate me, if I get angry, it's my responsibility. I think one of the greatest steps a parent can take is to ask for forgiveness from a child or spouse after he has lost his temper. All of us fail. The only real way to accept and correct the problem is to bring it out into the open and talk about it honestly.

This became a reality in my own life when I learned the concept that *God makes up the difference* from Ruth Carter Stapleton. When I came to realize I was not able to love my wife enough— that she needed more than I could give her—I began to pray that God would make up the difference in her life between the love I was giving her and the love she needed.

I talked to both my children about this and confessed I had never been able to give them all the love they needed in their growing years. I told them I was praying God would make the difference up to them.

This illustrates a basic principle that the ultimate in healing comes when we are able to face our inadequacies, see the hurt this causes others, and deal with these imperfections by being as honest as it is possible for us to be.

12

How to Heal Past Emotional Hurts

As I have shown, all of us have deep inner hurts, which come out of our relationships with other people and/or circumstances beyond our control. If these hurts are allowed to continue simmering below the surface, we develop symptoms and/or actual physical disease because of them. But how do we find healing for those deep, inner, lingering, emotional hurts?

Steps in Dealing With Disappointments

First, you must accept the fact that you will always have some disappointments in life. As long as you continue to expect perfection in all situations, you will have a somewhat unrealistic view of life. Denying there are problems is like trying to sweep dirt under the rug. All you end up with is a lumpy rug.

The facts of a life experience are undeniable, but the hurt feelings that come from these life events are very easily denied or suppressed. This is especially true when there is no apparent answer. The ego, the little self-god, the little child within us says, "It isn't so. It didn't happen. I don't want this hurt." We end up living in a state of self-deception—a state of nonreality. You have to accept that "there is a problem" before you can begin to correct it.

Second, you must face the fact of the hurt feelings or disappointment. Denying the emotional part of a problem is being dishonest to ourselves about our feelings. But when we accept these negative emotions, we can go on to experience a healing of these inner hurts. It is not always easy to control our emotions. Sometimes it is humanly impossible to control them. Remember, we're not perfect. But the fact that we cannot control whether or not a bird flies over our head is no reason to let it build a nest in our hair. So, too, with our emotions; we must accept them as the natural result of our relationships with others. As I look back on my own life, my deepest hurts and greatest disappointments have been my greatest growth experiences. As my pastor says, "There is no gain without pain." When we experience physical pain that is more than our nervous system can handle, we will faint or pass out. Likewise, when we experience an emotional hurt greater than our ability to cope, our mind will short-circuit the pain and suppress it into our subconscious.

But the suppression is not a long-term answer. Though it may be the only way to cope with the immediate shock to our emotions, it doesn't really deal with the problem; it merely postpones it. Suppressing emotional hurts deep inside is like putting the lid on a pressure cooker and turning up the burner. The pressure builds and will be expressed through our body one way or another. It may come out either in verbally expressed emotions or be diverted into dis—ease in the stomach, colon, heart, lungs, or elsewhere.

Third, and most importantly, I believe the answer to pent-up negative feelings is experiencing forgiveness. The Bible makes clear this truth in 1 John 1:9. "If we confess [that is to express, to get it out, to face the reality of the hurts and our negative feelings toward those hurts] our sins, He is faithful and righteous to forgive us our sins and to cleanse us from all unrighteousness."

We must face and confess our own negative reactions. If we have reacted in a negative way, then we must take the responsibility for it, no matter how logical and reasonable the self-justification of our feelings seems to be. When we doubt God, it's sin. When we do something that is unloving and unkind, that too is sin. We stand responsible. When we confess our doubt and unloving acts to God, He forgives and cleanses us. The problem *is* no more. He blots it out of His memory.

Can You Learn to Forgive?

A patient came to me who had high blood pressure, an ulcer (his stomach was in constant distress), and insomnia. This man's problems involved his old boss. He related to me that his former employer had promised him a significant salary, part ownership in the company, and a share of the profits from his work. But it turned out that he received only a low salary, which he had accepted because of all the promises. He received almost nothing, compared to what he had been promised and felt was justly his. This man had a severe hatred for this former employer who had betrayed and exploited him. His physical symptoms were all a manifestation of the bitterness and deep sense of injustice he felt.

I pointed out to this patient that *he* was the one who was suffering. "Your former boss is not hurting. *You* have the high blood pressure, the ulcers, and can't sleep. *You* are the one whose anxiety, tension, and depression levels are up. As long as you carry this hatred within your life, *you* are going to suffer.

"We all have weaknesses. We all bring upon ourselves many of the problems which come our way in life. But think of Jesus for a moment. Even though He never sinned, He was betrayed, deserted, falsely condemned, and crucified on a cross—the most excruciatingly painful death known to man. That was a very unloving act on the part of those who did it. But in the height of that experience He prayed, 'Father, forgive them, because they really don't understand what they're doing.'

"Your former employer, who has exploited you, violated God's laws, because God's law commands that we act lovingly to others. This man is blinded and consumed with his selfish greed, he really doesn't know what he's doing. Although he is probably feeling quite smug about how he pulled one over on you, he doesn't have any conception of the depth of pain he has caused not only you, but God. In winning he is really losing. Unless this sin is forgiven, he's going to suffer eternally for it. Your prayer and inner feelings should be that of pity. 'Father, forgive him. He doesn't really understand what he's doing.' "

Then, as I frequently do, I asked, "Would you really like to see that man go to hell?"

"Oh, no," he replied. "I really wouldn't." (Only once have I heard someone say yes to that question.)

When we can come to the point where we see the deep hurts in another person, when we can see he's perpetuating his own demise, then we can feel an empathy for that person. We can begin to feel sorrow for him. Then we can begin to pray, "Father, forgive him, because he doesn't really understand what he's doing." This kind of attitude brings with it a healing for the spiritual hurts that are rumbling around inside of us. The secret to this man's healing was forgiveness—being willing to ask God to forgive the one who had offended him—and thus to experience forgiveness himself.

What Happens If You Don't Forgive?

The above example illustrates what will happen to us if we do not learn to forgive others; that is, we must be willing to let God forgive them. The tension of the hurt will stay in our subconscious minds until we confess and release it. The longer we hang on to our hurts, the more they will be converted into physical problems and result in dis—ease. We're told, "See to it that no one comes short of the grace of God; that no root of bitterness springing up causes trouble, and by it many be defiled" (Hebrews 12:15). When we don't forgive, we become bitter, and bitterness will destroy us.

Jesus went even further in His condemnation of an unwillingness to forgive. He said if we do not forgive—that is, if we are not willing for God to forgive—we will not be able to enter heaven. " 'For if you forgive men for their transgressions, your heavenly Father will also forgive you. But if you do not forgive men, then your Father will not forgive your transgressions' " (Matthew 6:14, 15).

Jesus was concerned about our willingness to release others from our feelings of bitterness. We must remember that even though we "forgive" someone for their offense against us, that does not absolve them from their violation of God's laws. Because God is God, He made the rules and He is the only One who can truly forgive the offenses men have committed against Him.

We Can Overcome Those Hurts

Recently, I came to understand that there have been three major disappointments in my life. First, my Dad died when I was four. He had bad stomach ulcers and then developed pneumonia in the days before antibiotics. He didn't choose to die, but that didn't make my hurt any less painful. I had a large void and great disappointment in not having a dad.

Second, I'm disappointed in my mother. My mother was a wonderful Christian woman, but she had some very rigid "religious," ideals that bent me out of shape and gave me an odd-ball self-image early in life. When I was in the seventh grade, Walt Disney's *Snow White and the Seven Dwarfs* came to the local theater. Every child in grade school went to see that movie—except me. It was one of those "sinful things Christians can't do." The teacher who had to stay behind with me wasn't happy either. My mother meant well. She had her heart in the right place and was trying to do right for me, but it still hurt.

Third, I was disappointed with God. Why did He have to let my father die? Why did He permit my mother to be so "religious"? Deep within my subconscious was a feeling of bitterness toward God for allowing these things to happen to me. It wasn't until recently I was finally able to see the extent of my bitterness toward God and ask Him to forgive me. I have learned God knows what He is doing.

So, I have come to grips with my childish omnipotence, the little god within me, and say, "Okay, I'm going to accept the hurts that have come to me. But I don't have to remain the victim of them."

The Healing of Memories

The first, and most important way to heal emotional-spiritual hurts is to be willing to let God forgive the offender. The second factor is the healing of those bad experiences we have had in the past—to personally experience a "healing of memories."

What we are is the sum of all the experiences we have had up until this moment. And except for this moment, all that we are emotionally and mentally is memory. Unresolved hurts, stored in our memory, tend to create tensions and uneasiness within. Tension itself creates dis—ease and disease.

I was talking to a young woman with the usual nutritional problems of fatigue and stress. I asked her, "What was one of the biggest hurts that has happened to you?"

She stopped for a moment, then began to cry. "Well, it was when I was raped when I was twelve years old."

A person who assaults someone like that is sick; they certainly don't understand what they're doing. But that's why Christ was crucified, that we might have forgiveness. And in forgiveness is love and mercy and healing. Such memories can be healed.

What does Corrie ten Boom, the author of *The Hiding Place*, say? In her life she was a victim of the Nazis' atrocities. But she says, "Jesus is victor!" Just because we're victims doesn't mean we have to stay victims. We can become victors. Corrie certainly didn't stay a victim.

On another occasion, I asked the same question of a Christian woman. She replied, "Well, my mother and father used to argue a lot. I can remember one day in particular, when my mother took a butcher knife after Dad." She could still vividly remember the anger and the arguing and the conflict in her home. She could still feel the constant hostility, which eventually caused her father to leave.

She began to cry. Twenty-five years later, the memory of those hurts still brought tears to her eyes. It doesn't make any difference if you say, "It had to be," or "You were better off without him." It still hurts. She was without a dad and she could not fill that empty void by any other means.

I suggested we experiment with a healing-of-memories meditation. I had her relax, close her eyes, and visualize that scene again, as it had been twenty-five years ago. I asked her to feel the anger, the tension, the anxiety on her part. Now I said, "Be aware of the presence of Jesus—the warm, loving, kind presence of the Person of Jesus. Now watch that scene and let Jesus do what He wants to do. When you're done, tell me about it."

After a few minutes, she took a deep breath and opened her eyes. I asked, "What happened?"

"Well," she said, "as I watched, Jesus went over to my mother and took the butcher knife out of her hand. He took both mother and father in His arms and He loved them. Then He came over and held me." That's a healing of the memories. Only through a spiritual healing, through the divine intervention of Jesus, can such memories be healed.

A middle-aged woman came to me, distressed over her lack of empathy and feeling. She felt her emotions were dead in relation to her family. I questioned her about her early life and what might be causing this poor self-image and a very distinct lack of self-worth, which I had sensed in her. She didn't think she had any problem with her parents, but said, "I think it was with my peers. When I was a child, I had crooked teeth and badly crossed eyes; much worse than what I have now. I've had surgery to correct the eye problem and have had my teeth straightened. I can remember being teased about my eye problem and about my metal-rimmed glasses. The kids used to take my glasses away from me and break them. I can remember once they tied me up and made fun of me, breaking my glasses."

"Can you remember that incident?" I asked. "Can you visualize it in your mind?"

"Oh, yes, I certainly can."

I suggested she relax, put her hands in her lap, and visualize that event back in her youth. "Just act as though you are an observer and this is a scene that is being reenacted in front of you. Begin to feel the pain, the humiliation, the anger, the hurt that that little girl experienced. Feel the ropes, as they bound you in that past."

I paused for a few moments. "Now, I want you to become aware of another presence in that picture: the Person and the living presence of Jesus. Let Jesus do what He wants to do."

As she watched, Jesus went over to the little girl, untied and unwound the rope that was binding her. Then He picked the little girl up in His arms and carried her away.

Here's an illustration of a rather drastic hurt that occurred back in this patient's young life. The hurt was the result of something over which she had absolutely no control; the woman certainly had no choice in the creation of her vision and teeth problems. Her peers had printed on her mind a very negative self-acceptance picture.

This hurt had been deeply suppressed inside. At the time she was bound, she wasn't able to express her anger or react. It's probable she had never talked to anyone about this incident. It was one of the core reasons for her inability to express herself and be a warm part of her family.

Now thirty-five years later, through experiencing the healing of memories, she was able to release the hurt that had been simmering deep inside. First, she visualized this experience with some of the intensity with which it had happened. Then by allowing the timeless Christ to come into the picture, she was able to find healing and release. She was able to let her emotions go and set loose the ache which she had had bound up inside for so many years.

Dealing With a Past Problem

On my fifty-fourth birthday, I was thinking about my past and the death of my father fifty years before. As I reminisced, into my mind came the picture of a dark room, in which a small four-year-old boy—myself—lay sick in a big bed with what they then called "brain fever." I don't really know what I had, but it was probably some form of meningitis. I was quite sick.

As I watched, the door opened, and when the light poured into the room, my eyes throbbed with pain. The door closed and in a moment my mother slipped into bed beside me. Her presence helped me slip off into a quiet sleep. In a few days, I was recovered enough to go home with her.

As we entered the house, my mother stopped, knelt down beside me and said, "David, I have something to tell you. Daddy isn't here anymore. He's gone to be with Jesus."

I pulled myself away and went screaming off to the bedroom where my daddy had been. Throwing myself on the bed, I screamed, "I want my daddy! I want my daddy! I want my daddy!"

As I was seeing this picture in my mind, I sensed the presence of the strong, hairy-armed, loving Carpenter Jesus come into the room. I saw Him go over to the bed and pick up the little boy and hold him on His shoulder. As he patted the boy on the head, I heard Him say, "That's all right, David. I'll be your daddy from now on."

The actual experience happened fifty years ago, but the healing of my memory came just a year ago. Since that time, I've had a freedom within my inner self that I've never experienced before. There's been a filling of that void in my life, which I simply don't have any way of explaining. There is an inner peace, a sense of being loved, and really knowing that I am loved. Experiencing that love has brought a relief from the anger and bitterness I felt for all those years of not having a dad.

13
Total Inner Healing

Finding Peace of Mind

After I have completed my initial examination with most new patients, I ask, "Is there anything else?" When I asked this of one patient, he hesitated, started to say something, then stopped.

I encouraged him. "Go ahead, tell me what it is."

"Well," he said, "I would just like to have peace of mind."

"Peace of mind?" I replied. "I'm sure that isn't a false hope or an unrealistic desire. I'm certain it's possible for everyone to have peace of mind."

Previously, this patient had identified himself as having a religious background (even though he was not currently practicing his faith), so I wasn't hesitant about talking to him about God. I continued, "I'm certain peace of mind comes out of faith and trust in God.

"Faith is not something we're born with. It is something that must have a beginning in our lives. 'In the beginning God created the heavens and the earth.' There is one God, one Source, one Creator, and one Savior. It's difficult for us to put faith in an intangible 'something' that we cannot physically feel, see, or hear. But it is not impossible. We all put faith in intangible unexplainable concepts.

"For instance, what is this?" I asked drawing a number *1* on a prescription pad.

"The number one," he answered.

"Can you prove it?" I asked. He struggled a moment, trying with logic and reason to validate the concept of one.

"I guess it is a reality you can't prove."

Then I asked, "Do you believe your mother loves you?"

"Of course," he said.

"Can you prove to me she loves you?" Again he thought a moment, then replied he couldn't prove her love. He could have told me about things she does *because* she loves him, but those things do not *prove* her love.

"So, then, there are a number of intangible concepts and ideas that we cannot prove, yet we can know and put our faith and trust in them. The same is true with God. God is Someone we cannot prove, but we can come to the point of faith that accepts Him. If we accept the fact that 'God IS!' we have a positive concept; but if we question, 'Is God?' we are in a totally negative doubting position.

"Why is all this important to peace of mind? Because peace of mind comes out of a sense of faith and hope, rather than out of a sense of questioning and doubt. When we put our trust and faith in the concept that 'God is', and that He loves us, then we have the basis for true peace of mind. We have confidence not only in this life, but in the next life.

"The Bible says in 1 John 5:13, 'These things I have written to you who believe in the name of the Son of God, in order that you may know that you have eternal life.' This is the only basis for peace of mind."

This patient was looking at peace of mind as being only a mental state. It *is* a mental state, but that's just a part of it. True satisfying peace of mind comes from God. It is knowing that He is who He says He is; that He has done what He says He has done; and He will do what He says He will do.

We Can Know God

Man has a physical body, created from the dust of the ground. He has a spiritual soul, created in God's image. We have a dual entity: we are both physical and spiritual. It is the spiritual side of us that is able to know God. We can know God in the same sense that we can know the number *1*, or that "Mother loves us," or any other basically intangible concept.

The physical mind functions on a logical, rational basis and is constantly striving to *understand* what it knows. There is a vast difference between knowledge of something and understanding it. The telephone is a very important part of my life, but I do not have to understand all the intricate wires and computer components in the telephone system to enjoy its benefits. We probably do not understand 1 percent of all of the instruments and mechanical devices we use on a daily basis. It is not necessary that we understand the minute intricacies of all these tools. It is only important that we know how to use them properly.

This is true in our concept of God. We can know Him but we cannot understand Him. In the same sense we know we are loved by Him, even though we cannot fully understand and logically explain why. When I accept that God is; that He is love; that He loved me enough to send His Son Jesus to die on a cross for me; and that failing to be loving to other people is sin—*then* I have His peace of mind.

Once I become aware I have been alienated from God, I will know I need the sacrifice which Christ accomplished on the cross. Because of Christ's gift of His life for mine, I can be free from my sin. Freedom from sin comes through confession. If I confess I have sinned, then I can know God is faithful and just to forgive me and to cleanse me from all unrighteousness (1 John 1:9).

Faith in God is so utterly simple, it is hard to believe—and in turn, impossible to understand. Yet it is a fact, as affirmed by millions down through the centuries. When I fulfill the conditions that God asks—He has already done His part—then I receive His love. He loves me, even when I'm unloving; He forgives and cleanses me. It's that simple. God loved man enough to give His Son to die that we might live. This is an infinite spiritual fact, so utterly simple it is impossible for finite humans to understand.

Happily, it is not necessary to understand God's love. We can know without understanding. I know my wife loves me, but I do not understand how or why she does. I know God loves me based on my faith in His Word.

I attend our local Christian Businessmen's Committee breakfast, which meets every Tuesday morning. Recently I walked in and sat beside a man I thought was a stranger.

"You don't remember me, do you?" he said. "Several years ago I was a patient of yours. When I came to you, I was in the car-leasing business."

Slowly my memory chemicals began to be stimulated. "You said something to me that I'm sure helped save my life. When I came to you, I had a bad temper; I would blow off at the slightest provocation and I had roughed up several people quite badly. You showed me my poor diet was a major contributing factor.

"One day, as we were talking about me and my temper problem, you said, 'You know, Tony, they put people like you away. I think what you need is God.' That really made me mad. I never came back and wouldn't pay my bill."

By this time I could remember Tony quite clearly. "Yes. I remember you called me on the phone and yelled at me, saying, 'You claim to be such a good Christian and you sent me to collection! What kind of brotherly love is that!' I explained to you, at that time, that if I let you be dishonest—literally stealing from people—without trying to help you, I would be feeding your weaknesses and contributing to your problem. Jesus didn't go around pacifying people. He didn't compromise one widow's mite with the rich young ruler to keep him from turning away."

Tony continued. "Things went from bad to worse for me. I lost my leasing company; my wife and thirteen-year-old son left; I lost my home; I was fired from another job; and I was deeply in debt. I seriously considered suicide.

"Then one day my brother-in-law asked me to go to a Saturday-morning men's breakfast. There I heard a businessman share that he had been where I was then. But the love of Jesus Christ had transformed his life. He challenged us, if we didn't know Christ personally, to dare to believe He was the person He said He was. I had tried about everything else, so I decided to give Jesus a try. And Doc, you just can't imagine the changes in my life, since I dared to believe God. It all started back there when you told me, 'They put people like you away,' and 'God is your only hope.' "

We Must Meet His Conditions

Just as you can know the love of a parent or a wife or husband, in an even more real way, you can know God's love. When you come to the point where you say, "Hey, God, are You real? If You are, I want to know You. I'm going to dare to believe You are who You say You are. Please forgive me, as You have said You will do." Then it is God's responsibility to prove Himself true.

But in order to reach that point, we must come to the confession that "God, I'm a sinner. I've doubted You. I've failed to be loving." That's the barrier God will not cross. He will not force Himself upon us. It is only as we face our pride and the negative factors within our lives and confess them, that we find forgiveness and cleansing. And with that comes peace of mind.

Then you know *that you know that you know* that everything is right between you and God. Deep inside you hear His still small voice assuring you that He is there and that He loves you. To me the greatest awareness I have is "that Jesus loves me."

His love for us is the greatest love, because the greatest love involves giving your life for someone else. And Christ died on the cross. He was crucified for us. He rose again and He lives today. He lives in such a manner that, as He says in Revelation 3:20 (KJV), "Behold, I stand at the door, and knock: if any man hear my voice, and open the door, I will come in to him, and sup with him, and he with me." So when Christ comes into my life, He sits in the throne room of my inner self and becomes a part of me.

God Sets My Value

The developer or creator or owner of something has the right to establish its value. An artist sets the value on his painting or sculpture. A newspaper publisher decides the value of his daily paper. The farmer sets the price on his produce.

God knows us completely and perfectly. He created us in His own image. We are the last and the highest of His creations. God has the prerogative of establishing our value—of determining our worth. We do not. God set a value on mankind that was so high, it was worth it for Him to give His Son, so He could get us back.

I'm sure God's evaluation of my worth is far greater than what I could ever think or imagine. So if God loves and values me that much, and I accept His love and evaluation of me, then I can accept myself to be of *great value.* Who am I to belittle or reject God's evaluation? Isn't it a good feeling to know that you are that valuable in God's eyes?

I became a Christian very early in life, at age four. I grew up in a very religious world and went to a parochial high school and college. I was steeped in a religious environment, but it wasn't until I was forty years old that I came to understand the concept of self-love.

As I was reading the book *Self-Love* by my pastor, Dr. Robert Schuller, suddenly I became vividly aware that I could love myself *because God loved me.* Prior to that time, I had a lot of misgivings and self-doubt. I also had many rigid attitudes toward life that were very binding. Once I accepted the concept that God loved me and set my value, I was able to begin loving and accepting myself. I had had a great deal of difficulty with this "self-love" concept up to that time.

Self-Love Is Essential to Loving Others

In my practice, I have had more than 1,000 ministers and missionaries as patients. I find that these people often have a great struggle accepting this concept of self-love. Many are steeped with rigid religious doctrines that constrict them into narrow molds.

These molds say: "I am to be nothing. I must be a doormat, lowly, valueless. God doesn't need me." All of these concepts are antiscriptural and anti-Christian. They are an insult to God. If we are so valueless, why should God give His most valuable asset for us?

It is impossible to love others adequately, until I have learned to see myself as being *infinitely* valuable and, as such, I can learn to accept and love myself. The person who does not love himself, because God loves *him*, is actually a selfish, self-centered egotist. As a self-centered person, he is terribly insecure. He will constantly be searching to prove his worth. In focusing on his own little "self-god" within and his own selfish self-interests, he becomes extremely internalized. Therefore he cannot reach out adequately to love others.

The most basic spiritual-human principle is that of responsibility. I have to be responsible to and for myself, first. I am the only one who will have to answer to God for my choices. People with very rigid religious backgrounds or concepts find it is much easier to delegate the responsibility of self to someone else such as the church, or a set of rules, or to some leader. They become valueless "nothings" and tend to avoid facing the responsibility for their own lives and their own reactions.

My first responsibility is to love God. That's a responsibility I have to me; no one else can do it. When I choose to be and act responsible for me, then I set an example for others to see. If I put others above myself, then I give other people a sense that I am irresponsible.

My second responsibility is to love myself. This involves accepting God's analysis of my worth. Until I do that, I will not be able to reach out fully and love others the way He wants me to.

My third responsibility is to love and care for my children, Tere and Mona, and my wife, Ruthe. I believe I have a greater responsibility to them than to my patients or neighbors.

My fourth responsibility is to love and care about "others" (that is, my patients, neighbors, government leaders, and those throughout the world). Connected with this, I believe, is the concept that I have a responsibility to share God's love with the world. That includes being responsible and loving and compassionate to anyone with whom I come into contact. If I can be kind and compassionate, if I can care and share and show to that person the love of God—the love He wants them to see—that speaks much louder than the words I say.

Most "Love" Is Not Complete

All of us have the need to be loved. We need to be wanted, needed, accepted, approved, loved, and forgiven—unconditionally. It is impossible to receive all the love we need on a human level, but that's where each of us starts.

Unfortunately, much of the *love* in the world is self-centered. It's centered on getting, rather than on giving. When a person does or gives something just to fill a personal need, his motive is selfish and self-centered. Such a motive basically is trying to buy love, attention, and acceptance. This is called greed giving and, in my opinion, is not true giving at all.

Need giving is when we give to help meet the needs of another person. This kind of giving is very constructive. Jesus talked about the essence of this kind of giving when He said, "If you save your life, you lose it" (*see* Matthew 16:25). On the opposite side of the coin is "If you give your life, then you save it." By feeling the hurts of others and reaching out and giving of ourselves to help fill their needs, we have our own needs for love fulfilled.

Turning Hurts Into Love

By nature, love is vulnerable. It is open, tender, fragile, and weak. Thus, to love someone is to make ourselves vulnerable to being hurt. At an early age most of us tried to express love to someone and were rejected. Usually that rejection was temporary or partial. But experiencing the pain of rejection conditions us to fear being rejected in the future. The human response to hurt is to react reflexly. Whether it is physical or emotional pain, we tend to automatically pull away and protect ourselves. When we reach out in pity or compassion to another person and that person responds in anger, our immediate reaction is to withdraw.

We tend to focus on *our pain* rather than on the hurt that caused the other person to react in anger. Pain is a more dominating feeling than pleasure. Physical and emotional pain paralyzes. It causes an acute focus on the problem. We want relief *now*.

Paradoxically, love is of great value in treating those who have severe chronic pain. In the Pain Clinic at the UCLA Medical Center, there is a standing order on many charts. The patient is to receive four hugs a day. The *laying on of hands* from one person to another has a loving, warm, compassionate, and therapeutic effect. It has major benefits to a person who is in a chronic pain state.

I was counseling a young man who was having a difficult time finishing high school. He was quite withdrawn and was having problems communicating, even with his peers. He gave the impression of being quite bound-up emotionally, so I asked about his homelife.

He said he had good relations with his mother but did quite poorly with his father, a cold, distant man, who didn't communicate well with anyone in the family. He couldn't remember ever hearing his father say, "I love you."

"Did you know your father's parents?"

"Oh, yes. They were from the old country; they were rigid, gruff, and short-spoken just like my father."

"That's interesting," I said. "Your father probably never learned how to express himself and give love to his family, because his parents were not the type of people who could teach him. Love needs to be taught. I would guess that deep inside, your father is hurting because he would *like* to express his love and concern to you, but he can't—because he's never learned how."

My young patient reflected for a few moments, then said, "Yeah . . . I wonder how I could help him." His answer was really the beginning of an answer to his own problems. Once one truly learns to reach out in love, his whole life will change for the better.

God Wants Us to Love, Even If It Hurts

According to Jesus, the second greatest commandment is to love others as much as we love ourselves. So when we are unloving to someone, we are violating God's law. To be truly loving means we must love in spite of the hurts others may inflict upon us.

A person who reacts in an unloving way is defensively expressing the hurts in his own life. There needs to come a time when we look at other people's behavior and see beyond their immediate reactions—when we try to see *why* they are acting in an "unloving" way! I'm certain most aggressive behavior can be traced back to not having been loved enough!

Being loved is a supportive, maturing, and positive building factor in our lives. The only real way we can be loved in the mature adult stage is to give love. This must be done without reservation. We can not qualify our love with an "I'll love you, if you love me" attitude. Love is based completely on free choice. It cannot be bought or coerced. It can't be legalized, tricked or beguiled. It can only be given out of free will.

That's the reason God gave us a free will. He wanted us to have the freedom to accept or reject His love. God will never force us to love Him. He could only give us the choice. What we do with His love is the beginning of learning to love others; it is also the beginning of all inner healing.

IV
Dealing With Specific Problems

14
Dealing With Extra Weight

The Sickness of Being Overweight

Ask the average overweight person how he feels, and he will undoubtedly say, "Oh, I'm fine." He doesn't think of himself as being sick; he doesn't have cancer, or pneumonia, or a broken leg; he's just overweight. That's a condition and not an illness in the minds of most people.

But being overweight is as much a sickness as having diabetes, arthritis, or hardening of the arteries. Obesity tends to shorten people's lives. It complicates high blood pressure, heart trouble, diabetes, and all other diseases. If we look at obesity as a sickness—a state of not being well—it is easier to deal with the problem. As long as the grossly overweight person thinks, "There is nothing wrong with me but my weight," he is in trouble.

A lady came to me recently who was five-foot-one, and weighed 250 pounds. Her initial request was, "I just want to lose weight, because I don't feel good this way." She had been overweight for twenty-five years. My experience tells me a person who is this obese for that long needs a radical change in her life. I didn't believe she could do it without help, so I put her in the hospital and fasted her, just to show her she could live and feel good without eating.

The results of my evaluation showed she was also significantly diabetic. She had no awareness she was diabetic. Without laboratory tests, there is no way she would have known she had the disease.

In the quiet, directed atmosphere of her hospital bed, she was able to do a lot of thinking about herself and come to grips with the fact that she was quite sick. She realized that if she didn't turn this problem around now, she never would. Her overall life-style had to change dramatically in order to control her diabetes and lose those excess pounds.

The Basic Problem

Overweight problems are 99 44/100 percent due to overeating. There are a few exceptional individuals whose glands are grossly malfunctioning. These unfortunates end up tipping the scales at four, five, or six hundred pounds. But for the most part, extra weight comes from extra food.

If we were to take all fat people and put them on a prolonged fast with adequate nutrients, they would lose weight. But keeping the extra pounds off is a very different situation.

The obese person who gains his weight after adolescence has greatly enlarged fat cells; he has not increased their number, only their size. Relatively speaking, his fat cells go from pint to quart size. The person who becomes obese before adolescence has the additional problem of having a greater number of fat cells as well.

A problem comes when a person loses weight; the cell walls do not shrink immediately to compensate for the new smaller quantity of fat. The cells look like small balloons, which have been blown up for some time. When they are deflated, they have a "stretched-out" appearance.

About 55 to 60 percent of our body is water; it is an integral part of all tissues. So it is common for fat cells that have lost a portion of their fat to swell up with water. (*See* Illustration I.) This is one of the reasons why you may lose fat, that is, body dimensions but still maintain the same body weight for a short time. It takes time for the walls of these cells to shrink back to normal size.

normal fat cell

 enlarged fat cell

 weight-loss fat cell

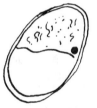 weight-loss fat cell
filled with water

Illustration I

There is an active mechanism within the body that tends to promote storage of energy carbohydrates into fat rather than utilize them. We see this in bears. They eat a tremendous amount through the summer and get fat. Then they hibernate during the winter and burn up that fat.

The problem with human beings is that once we have adapted our metabolism so that there is an increased fat production, we tend to maintain that kind of metabolism. It is difficult to revert back to a normal metabolism, which uses up carbohydrates rather than the type that tends to store them as fat.

Reducing Your Food Intake

So how do you go about reducing your food intake? First, you must think back to your early eating habits. This is where most obesity usually begins. It starts with your mental programming. How many times, as a child, were you told, "Clean up your plate"? Or how many times did you not have enough to eat, causing a deep fear of going hungry? Or how many times were you bribed to be good, with offers of food, or punished by the withholding of food?

So many mothers felt guilty if their children did not eat something—anything—even if it was totally unnourishing. They kept stuffing food into us to make us healthy. There used to be a concept that a fat baby was a healthy baby. We must realize this was a mistaken ideal. It doesn't hurt a child to miss a meal now and then. A slender child is usually much more healthy than a fat one.

Eating, besides being physically pleasing and satisfying, has many social and emotional benefits as well. Psychology speaks of "oral gratification," such as kissing, smoking, and sucking; we find pleasure in putting things into our mouths. Our eating is related as much to emotional satisfaction as it is to our need for nutrition. The social factors of "going out to eat" at restaurants, banquets, and parties are an everyday pleasantry. Most of the foods served are fat promoting versus fat reducing. So the social-emotional factors in obesity are considerable. The inner craving for love can easily be confused with a craving for food. Here again, I have found both personally and in my practice that a good "healing of the memories" helps significantly in controlling the appetite of a binge eater.

Most people with an obesity problem are heavy starch, fat, and sugar eaters. They have been programmed into eating this kind of food since childhood. By changing your tastes from high to low starch foods, like vegetables, grains, legumes, and low-calorie fruits—and restricting fats and oils—you can drastically reduce your caloric intake, increase bulk, and improve elimination. All of these things tend to promote better nutrition and to normalize your weight.

A Lifetime Problem

Dealing with obesity is a lifelong problem. It is only controlled—never cured. Weight loss begins in the mind, not at the dinner table, or at the take-out window. An obese person must have a deep desire to change his eating habits—if he is to lose weight on a permanent basis.

Research has been done on mice that were litter mates. One group was fed twice a day; the other group was allowed to nibble all day long. By the time they reached maturity, those who nibbled all day long were of normal weight, while those who had eaten twice a day were two or three times heavier than the nibblers.

A person who is overweight often thinks, "I must cut back." So he starts skipping meals. Unfortunately, this usually causes him to gain even more weight. When he does eat, he eats heavier meals, because he is hungrier.

You are much better off eating small amounts of food frequently; that tends to satisfy the hunger problem. You don't get as hungry, so you eat less. I've had many patients on six small feedings a day who say, "I just never get hungry. I have to think to take my snacks."

To achieve and maintain a slim, trim, happy-with-yourself you, the basic need is to learn to eat right and have an adequate weight-controlling exercise program. Eat foods that are high in fiber, bulk, complex carbohydrates, and protein servings totaling sixty grams a day. Avoid, without exception, high-carbohydrate, high-fat and refined foods.

I should mention here a recent study by three University of Cincinnati medical-school psychologists. They feel it is emotionally and/or metabolically impossible for some grossly overweight people to lose weight. For these few, a rigidly strict (and tormenting) diet may be more stressful than living with the problem the best they can. For those unfortunate few, I agree, and I am sorry for them.

Become More Active

Another important factor in weight loss is physical activity. Recent studies show that overweight people often eat *less* than slim people of the same age group. The big difference is that those who are slimmer are much more active and burn up more of their caloric intake.

If you want to lose weight, and you do not have a good exercise and physical fitness program, reread chapter 9 and become more physically active. This will go a long way toward helping you control your weight problem.

Overcoming Discouragement

One of the difficulties in getting to be the "slim and trim you" is the problem of discouragement. We live in a day when everything is instant. We've been negatively programmed to believe that weight loss can come quickly—almost magically—and if it doesn't, we're not doing something right. After all, Mr. and Mrs. Fat-Turned-Slim in the TV commercial or the magazine ad did it painlessly, while eating everything they wanted—all in just one month! We are brainwashed into believing that weight loss can be almost instantaneous and completely painless.

Four to six pounds a month is the average for most patients on a good "slim and trim" program. In the initial stages, if a person is quite heavy, he may lose faster, but there comes a time in which the rapid weight loss doesn't happen regularly. In fact, you may plateau and not lose anything for six to eight weeks.

When this happens, you have to look at your life in terms of your total future perspective, rather than become discouraged because you aren't losing as fast as you had imagined. Most of the time we use the "scale" as the only measuring device to determine progress. If we don't see results, we become discouraged. But as with all life cycles, you will lose weight for a while, plateau, then lose weight again.

Fat has much more volume per pound than does muscle. As you begin to eat right and increase your physical-activity level, you will lose flab and build muscle tone. For this reason, your weight may not drop but your bust, waist, and hip size will.

I had a patient recently who became extremely discouraged because she had plateaued, after moving from 260 to 225. "Nothing's happening," she said. "I haven't lost any weight for two or three months." I went back through her charts and looked at her measurements, which we recorded each visit. I found that during this period she had lost three inches in the bust, seven inches in the waist, and three inches in the hips. Although she hadn't lost weight, she had changed dress sizes without realizing it.

When I asked her how her clothes were fitting, she admitted, "I am getting into clothes I haven't been able to wear for a long time."

A great benefit can also be obtained through group participation in a weight-loss program. Weight Watchers, Over-Eaters Anonymous, and other such organizations can give you the positive reinforcement and encouragement you need.

You have to be willing to swallow your pride and the childish idea, "I can do it myself." Take whatever time and effort is necessary to reach your goal. It is a matter of knowing what you have to give up in order to get ahead. You have to feel the benefits of losing your excess weight are sufficient to make the struggle and suffering worthwhile.

Program Your Mind

Obese people are self-haters. They think of themselves as ugly. They need to begin loving themselves, seeing what God sees, and accepting themselves as He does.

"Then why," you may ask, "did God let me get this way?" Remember, He did not create you this way. Sin and sickness came into this world because Adam and Eve chose to doubt, rebel, and disobey. They chose to listen to Satan's lies. Your sickness came about because of the evil Satan brought into the world, not because God was trying to be mean or punish you.

The success of a weight-loss program lies, first, in changing your thinking. Changing your thinking is done through: (1) believing it can be done; (2) positive affirmations; and (3) mental conditioning. Proverbs says, "As a man thinketh in his heart, so is he" (*see* Proverbs 23:7). The programming of our thinking determines how we feel, act, and are. A person who is grossly overweight is that way, unless he or she is the exception with a glandular problem, because that's how he's been programmed to think and eat. So it is necessary to change the pattern of that deep inner thinking.

We can change our thinking by saying a positive affirmation every day. This should be done two times a day—once in the morning and once in the evening. By doing this on a rote basis, consistently, it will change your deep inner thinking. An example of an affirmation is: *It feels so good to feel good without all those fats, starches, and sickening sweets. There is a beautiful person deep inside of me that God loves and accepts now, just as I am.* Say it, or a similar statement, over and over, without trying to force yourself into changing. Do it, without interruption, for twenty-one days in a row, and you *will* change your deep inner thinking.

Remember, whenever there is an element of doubt, you are less able to do what you want to do. But God doesn't want you to struggle, fret, and wring your hands, trying to force yourself into new rigid, negative behavior. You can do it naturally and easily by the consistent, abstract, "inch by inch, anything's a cinch," repetitive reprogramming of your attitudes and behavior. This will build new and positive thought patterns in your inner computer.

15
Hypoglycemia and Diabetes

The Hypoglycemia Problem

"Hypo" means *below;* "glycemia" means *sugar in the blood stream.* There is a lot of confusion and misunderstanding about this highly symptomatic condition. In classical medicine, there are those who belligerently reject hypoglycemia as a concept. Others accept it, but say that the blood sugar must drop below 50 milligram percent in order for the patient to have a hypoglycemic problem.

In my opinion, it really doesn't matter how low or how high the blood sugar gets (within limits) during a blood-sugar test. A diagnosis of hypoglycemia is made on how the patient reacts during the test. The numbers on the laboratory test are only important if they run well above or below the normal range. And hypoglycemia is only a part of the sugar problem.

Many people are very sensitive to sugar and/or the chemicals used to process it. When they eat something with even a small amount of sugar in it, they get a reaction. It may be weakness, tremors, the shakes, cold sweats, rapid heartbeat, palpitations, headache, dizziness, anxiety, nausea, stomachache or cramps, confusion, light-headedness, depression, and so on. These people are sick, whether you call the problem hypoglycemia, sugar sensitivity, or something else. If you have this problem, you are, first, physically sick; then, second, emotionally, neurotically or psychotically sick.

Sugar Sneaks Up on Us

Most of the time, the sugar we eat is hidden in our foods. Sugar comes in many forms, with many names: syrup, glucose, sucrose, brown sugar, fructose, corn sweetener, molasses, turbinado sugar, caramel, and dextrose. Probably 70 to 75 percent of the foods available in our grocery markets have sugar in them. Even many natural-appearing foods unsuspectingly contain large amounts of sugar. We can also get a heavy dose of sugar from a natural source such as orange juice. Here the sugar's form has been released from solid fibrous segments to a liquid. The free sugar is instantly available for absorption into the body.

I had a patient once who would drink a quart of orange juice at one sitting, and then he would develop a number of the sugar overload symptoms mentioned above. That quart of juice probably contains 100 to 130 grams of sugar. Just because you are eating an orange from a natural source, doesn't mean you may not be overloading your body with sugar. Again, the key is, what are your symptoms? You must listen to your body. It will tell you if you are reacting to sugar, or milk, or wheat, or whatever.

Don't be fooled or ridiculed by others. If you eat or drink or breathe something and it repeatedly makes you feel bad in some way, trust your senses. The other person may not react to what makes you sick. *You're* the one that's feeling the symptoms. Accept and trust yourself as being the most knowledgeable person as to how good or how bad you feel.

I have many patients who have recovered from their depressions, phobias, hallucinations, quick-temperedness, tired, weak feelings, loss of energy, acute anxiety, headaches, and sleeplessness by avoiding all foods containing sugar and the other refined carbohydrates. By changing their diets and adding high-dosage levels of vitamins, minerals, and amino acids, they have improved dramatically. (This process of renewal usually takes three to four months. It took the body a long time to get into that depleted state, and recovery isn't something that will happen to you in a day or a week.)

In hypoglycemia and/or sugar sensitivity, the person feels sick. It's difficult for them to live with the sickness until the body is able to renew itself. They feel so bad they want something done *now*. But, again, *it takes time*, usually three to four months, or longer, for the renewal process to take place.

The usual course of recovery is up and down. The patient will feel good one day, and down the next. They will feel depressed and anxious, because they think they aren't getting well. They will need to stick to their strict, no-refined carbohydrate diet. Again, many hypoglycemics have multiple food allergies. These two problems must be thought of together and often are combined in treatment.

Sugar sensitivity and/or hypoglycemia is not an organic disease, as are appendicitis, gallstones, and cancer. It is a metabolic condition of imbalance. When the body is fed the proper nutrients to restore it to its optimum function, the symptoms that result from the depletion caused by taking in too much sugar and/or other refined carbohydrates can be controlled. Then the body will function normally. This is a malady that is never cured, only controlled.

The Diabetic Problem

The opposite side of *hypo*glycemia is *hyper*glycemia or diabetes, as it is commonly known. There are many forms of diabetes, most of which can be controlled through a proper eating and exercise regimen. The diet of a hypoglycemic and a diabetic are nearly identical. They both need to avoid refined carbohydrates and fats. They need to eat "little and often." They need to learn that diet is the primary way of controlling their problem.

A hypoglycemic overproduces insulin for a short period of time. That drives the blood sugar down. A diabetic doesn't produce enough insulin to keep the blood-sugar levels down to normal. In this condition the blood sugar goes up and stays up for an extended period of time.

Some people are born with a relatively small number of beta cells in their pancreas. (These are the cells that produce insulin.) Others are born with maybe a hundred times more. The person who has just a few of these cells is more susceptible to wearing them out quickly, or to having an infection which destroys them quickly. So any stress that tends to overstimulate the beta cells of the pancreas (whether it's a viral disease or overuse) tends to wear out and reduce the gland's ability to produce insulin and the body's ability to control its blood sugar.

The Glucose Tolerance Test

A glucose tolerance test is the standard test to determine both hypoglycemia and diabetes. I use a five-hour, eight specimen test. A blood sample is taken before the glucose challenge, then at ½-1-2-3-3½-4 and 5 hours. (*See* specimen forms in Appendix D.) I do not feel that a six-hour test is really necessary. In my experience, perhaps only 1 or 2 percent of patients will show a reaction and/or symptoms after the fifth hour.

However, 10 to 15 percent of abnormal hypoglycemic curves will show their maximum drop and symptoms at 3½ hours after the test begins. Most labs only draw speciments at 0-½-1-2-3-4 and 5 hours. They do not take a specimen at 3½ hours. So they miss the time many people show truly positive hypoglycemic blood-sugar levels.

Another thing I look for is how rapidly the blood-sugar level drops. If the sugar level drops more than 50 milligram percent in an hour, that is considered to be due to the overproduction of insulin. But—again—the final diagnosis is determined by how the patient reacts.

During testing I have had patients who have nearly gone into shock. They have had profuse sweating, rapid heartbeat, shakes, extreme pallor, and other dramatic symptoms. Amazingly, at the time the test was suspended, the blood-sugar levels are sometimes still in the normal range. Obviously, your symptoms tell much more than the numbers on the blood-sugar curve.

Diet Suggestions

The basic diet recommendations for hypoglycemics and diabetics are: one, avoid all refined carbohydrates; two, avoid a high intake of fats and oils (15 to 20 percent of your caloric intake is more than enough); three, eat small amounts of food frequently (five or six times a day is best); and, four, take adequate supplements. The supplements I feel these two diseases need are substantial amounts of the vitamin B complex (50 milligram range), a good hydrolyzed amino acid complex, and a mineral supplement that includes all of the minerals, but especially magnesium, chromium, and zinc.

Eating only once or twice a day or overindulging in refined carbohydrates and fats is hazardous; such bad habits create tremendous control problems in both these diseases. There is evidence that many adult diabetics have gone through a hypoglycemic stage. But it is *not true* that all hypoglycemics become diabetics. Some of them do, but most of them don't, particularly those who learn how to control their diets and take the proper supplements.

A diabetic often benefits greatly by fasting one or two days a week. I believe a diabetic learning to fast *must be supervised by a physician.* A diabetic who has a markedly high blood sugar and/or overt diabetic symptoms or has ketosis could get himself into serious trouble by trying a thirty-hour fast on his own. If this is your situation, *do not try it without expert help.*

16
Nutrition in Pregnancy

Nutrition in pregnancy should begin at least six months, if not a year, *before* a woman plans to become pregnant. Once pregnancy starts, the growing embryo places tremendous demands on the nutritional reserves in a woman's body. So many chemical changes take place, that it is difficult for a woman to catch up, if she doesn't have a good reserve already on hand. If she is depleted before beginning pregnancy, she will in all probability end up even more depleted nine months later.

The first three months are the most important period in the intrauterine growth process. It is in the first three months that protein and vitamin deficiencies, as well as toxic reactions to drugs and other chemicals, have their most detrimental effect. It is during the first trimester that infections such as German measles can cause birth defects. Any congenital malformation occurring at this time will remain with the child for life.

The nutritional stores in a woman's body and her food intake are the only source of vitamins, minerals, proteins, and energy the fetus has. They must be present in the mother's body in optimum amounts, so that she can provide all the fetus needs to be a healthy baby. If she doesn't have them, the baby will suffer.

For these reasons, pregnancy should be planned nutritionally well in advance of conception. The expectant mother should begin eating optimally and taking added supplements six to eight months *before* she plans to get pregnant. Waiting until after she has missed a period and going to a doctor for verification of her pregnancy is too late to begin an optimum nutritional program for both mother and child; but of course, it is far better to begin late than not to begin at all.

Nutrition during pregnancy is important. Review chapter 5 and religiously avoid junk foods, refined carbohydrates, and so on. Taking 60 to 100 milligrams of zinc a day will help prevent stretch marks. Extra calcium and magnesium are needed for bone formation. Additional folic acid and iron are necessary to avoid anemia in the mother. High doses of B^6 (pyridoxine), 100 to 600 milligrams a day, may alleviate morning sickness. I recommend purchase of a good book on nutrition in pregnancy and following a healthy diet as described in chapter 5.

The *don'ts* during pregnancy are as important as the *dos*. Avoid alcohol and cigarettes. Avoid over-the-counter drugs, unless they are approved by your physician and/or your pharmacist. (Pharmacists often have more information about drug side effects than physicians.) If you think you're pregnant and are on a medication for another problem, always check with your doctor to see if there are any reasons for discontinuing the medication. For example, if you are taking tetracycline to treat your acne, continued use of this antibiotic would probably cause deep yellow-orange stains in your baby's teeth.

It's okay to gain weight during your pregnancy, unless you are grossly overweight to begin with. I had one overweight patient, who started her pregnancy at 175 pounds. At full term she weighed 174 and delivered a normal baby. But that took a lot of careful supervision.

Fifteen to twenty pounds of weight gain is normal. Any less and you may have an underweight baby. Infants who are under "optimum weight" have many more survival problems than normal-weight babies.

17
Headaches

What Are Your Headache Symptoms?

There are many different kinds of headaches. If you were to come to me with a headache problem, the first question I would ask you is "How many kinds of headaches do you have?"

Many people have two or three or even four different kinds of headaches. They say, "One kind is over my eyes and is a steady pressure pain. Another is a pounding, throbbing pain in my right temple. And the third starts as a steady ache in the back of my head, then moves up over the top of my forehead. It usually becomes a severe, throbbing headache."

Next I ask, "Where do your headaches occur (where they happen geographically). Do you have them in the shower? At work? In the garage? Where?"

"What brings on your headaches?" Often, I have a patient keep a headache diary along with his diet diary. This is important, as it often provides the best clues for diagnosis.

"Does it throb and pound, or is it a steady dull ache? Is it a sharp, piercing pressure pain? Is it on one side of your head only? Does it alternate sides, or is it on both sides at the same time? Does it ever debilitate you (that is, make you stop work and cause you to lie down)? What relieves it? Aspirin, food, a manipulative treatment, or something else? Do you know why you get headaches?" Many people have a good idea why their headaches occur. It is important to ask for their opinion. A headache without a diagnosis is impossible to treat correctly.

The Different Kinds of Headaches

There are several different types of headaches. First, is the *tension* or *muscle-spasm* headache. I'm convinced all headaches have a muscle-spasm component. But in the tension headache, tight, tender muscles are the main problem. This type of headache could be caused by an injury, even twenty to thirty years ago. A rear-end auto accident or falling down some stairs could cause such headaches. Pressure on the job or marital conflict can bring on a tension headache. Chemical and allergy problems are also causes.

I have had many patients with early-morning headaches. I ask such people, "What type of pillow do you sleep on? What is it made of?" I have had at least a hundred patients who have had headaches due to sleeping on foam-rubber pillows. The stiffness and resilience of the foam rubber is enough to cause the neck and head to vibrate constantly causing tension and muscle spasms.

Second is the *sinus* headache. They can be due to breathing chemicals or pollens in the air. Fumes such as volatile petro-chemicals (soaps, gasoline, sprays, natural gas, perfumes, and smog) can cause this problem. An infection in your sinuses can also bring on this type of headache. A sinus headache is located in the face and forehead. It gets worse when bending the head down.

Third, are *vascular* headaches. The origin of this kind of headache is in the blood vessels of the neck and head. These are pounding, throbbing, and acutely debilitating headaches of the migraine or cluster type. My experience is that vascular headaches are of many causes, but most of the time there is an allergic and/or a nutritional and/or a musculo-skeletal factor contributing to the vascular problem.

Several years ago I was at a headache symposium in San Diego, California. A supposedly classic migraine-headache patient was presented along with her workup and treatment. After the lecture, I sought out the patient and asked, "Has anyone ever felt your neck?" She stopped and thought a moment, then said she could not remember that anyone ever had. "May I?" I asked. With her permission, I felt her neck and found several acutely tender, hard areas of muscle spasm. She wasn't aware of any neck problem, though she had had a back injury in the past.

It is important to know that, *in all headaches* (with rare exceptions) *there is a muscle-tension component.* My training as an osteopath has oriented me to look for musculo-skeletal structural problems. I find few headache patients, even those with migraine headaches, who do not have a significant amount of palpable muscle spasm and tenderness.

Almost universally I find there are great benefits from manipulative therapy for all types of headache problems. This is especially true if the patient has had headaches over a long period of time. Every muscle, tendon, ligament, and joint structure has a built-in memory of what is normal. Through a sprain, strain, or injury, this memory print can be changed to an abnormal "normal" which may last for years. Through manipulation techniques, often the memory can be changed back to a "normal" normal.

A fourth kind of headache are those of *organic origin*. These include those caused by a tumor, meningitis, or a stroke, and so forth.

Treating the Headache With Diet

Most of the patients who come to me with a headache problem think headaches just come on for no reason. But all headaches have a reason or a cause. People seldom think about foods and/or chemicals as the cause, because most people eat without thinking about what they are eating.

Food-related headaches are of two types. First, are the headaches that are caused by food allergies and/or chemical sensitivities. These usually come on after eating. Second, are those headaches that come on from going too long without food. This type of headache is related to a low blood sugar, tension, stress, and the "burn-out" problem.

There are many foods known to cause headaches. MSG (monosodium glutamate) is a well-known chemical that precipitates headaches. Someone noticed that every time he went to a Chinese restaurant, he developed a headache halfway through the meal. A little personal detective work revealed that the first course is almost always soup. A common flavor enhancer in Chinese foods, particularly in the soups, is monosodium glutamate.

Other headache-inducing foods and chemicals are sugar, caffeine, herb teas, chocolate, nitrites (as in ham, bacon, and luncheon meats), yeasts, nuts, lima bean pods, navy beans, sweet pod peas, onions, garlic, bananas, avocados, canned figs, chicken livers, and alcoholic drinks (particularly beer, red wines, and gin).

Foods that have been aged, fermented, pickled, or marinated are a frequent cause of headaches. These include vinegar, sour cream, aged cheeses (Cheddar, blue, Roquefort, and Camembert), and fresh, hot breads.

If you have recurrent headaches, keep a headache and diet diary for two or three weeks. See if you can find a food or chemical additive that may be bringing on your headaches. To be certain, try that food or chemical all by itself. With some substances, there may be a delayed response (that is, drinking red wine or gin at night results in waking up with a headache the next morning).

Some headache patients need help in multiple areas. One patient who came to me was quite depressed and had severe headaches. She had actually been placed in a mental institution for these problems. When I felt the back of her neck and head, she cringed with pain. "What did you do? That was so painful! I've never had anyone touch my neck like that before."

This woman's diagnostic evaluation included a hypoglycemic test—which was very positive. Her fast and food tests revealed she was also allergic to many foods. I placed her on a hypoglycemic diet and eliminated the foods to which she was allergic; I also prescribed high-potency supplements and muscle relaxants. Then I gave her physiotherapy and manipulative treatments. Within three months, she estimated 80 to 90 percent of her headache and depression problems had disappeared.

18
Strokes and Hardening
of the Arteries

It is true that people with high blood levels of cholesterol and/or triglycerides (natural fats) and/or sugar have a much higher incidence of atherosclerosis or hardening of the arteries. However, those of us in Wholistic Medicine believe it is the intake of refined carbohydrates, soft and hard fats, hydrogenated oils, and excessive fat and oil that are the real culprits.

In my opinion, this disease process is also brought on primarily by toxic substances and/or nutritional deficiencies in the diet. This is another civilization disease and is seldom seen in people who have natural food diets. Heart attacks, strokes, gangrene, and the other atherosclerotic diseases are responsible for more deaths in the United States than any other cause.

During the Vietnam conflict, autopsy examinations on American soldiers revealed that many of these men, even those in their early thirties, were beginning to develop calcium deposits on their blood-vessel walls.

Nathan Pritikin, at his Longevity Center in Santa Monica, California, has done extensive research on this subject. His findings show that reduction of the above list of food substances in our diets, plus exercise, dramatically reduces, and at times even reverses, this degenerative process.

All of us can have healthier bodies by avoiding salt, refined carbohydrates, and fats (particularly hydrogenated fats). Shortening, margarine, and nondairy creamers are oils that have been hydrogenated (that is changed from a liquid into a soft solid). You will find that these soft solid fats become liquid at a higher temperature (105 degrees) than normal body temperature. I am of the opinion that butter (which melts at 98 degrees) is much better for our bodies because it digests more quickly and comes from a more natural source. It also is a liquid at body temperature. It also tastes better!

Heart attacks and strokes, for the most part, are due to hardening or clogging of the arteries from increased calcium and cholesterol deposits in the walls of blood vessels. The arteries in diabetics may have this happen in the extremities. They may develop gangrenous toes or fingers, which may necessitate amputation. Diabetics also are prone to hardening of the blood vessels in the eye, which can cause blindness. Hardened arteries can cause a multitude of different diseases, all related to poor or obstructed circulation.

I believe an ideal program to prevent the diseases caused by clogging of the arteries is to improve both your diet and exercise. Completely avoid refined carbohydrates. Consume few fats and oils, avoiding the hard fats completely. Eat moderate amounts of protein (sixty to seventy grams a day in two servings is adequate). In addition, I recommend an exercise period of at least forty-five minutes at a time, three to four times a week.

19
Hypertension

There are two kinds of hypertension: organic and essential. Organic hypertension is due to some pathological process going on in the body, such as kidney disease, adrenal tumors, high thyroid, lead poisoning, and so forth. These are medical problems which should be cared for by your family physician.

Essential hypertension means that we in the medical profession don't really know what causes it. It is my personal opinion that this type of high blood pressure is primarily an emotional-spiritual problem. Both essential and organic hypertension have devastating physical effects.

Hypertension as a Spiritual-Emotional Problem

I believe that people with essential hypertension get caught up in a hectic, uncontrolled life-style. They don't take time to be themselves; they're always marching to the beat of someone else's drum. Consequently, they develop a deep inner anger and resentment, because they feel they are trapped and not able to be themselves. They get angry at themselves for feeling they must live up to a lot of "got tos" drummed into them by their parents and peers, so that they can be good enough and acceptable. Guilt complexes imposed on them by other people also make them angry and resentful. This usually starts in infancy and many people never free themselves from this mental bondage.

Whenever anything fearful or life threatening happens, our adrenaline instantly flows, shooting up our pulse and blood pressure. As I often say to my patients, "If there was a sudden explosion in this building, and it was followed by a roaring fire, we wouldn't need to stop and hold a committee meeting to decide what to do. We'd all be on our way outside without scarcely thinking about it."

All mankind, since the Fall, has been born with the inherited weaknesses of fear and worry. As I have previously written, the fear of death and the unknown is a deep concern and anxiety in all of us. It is a negative internal pressure that is constantly present. It is less obvious than the fear which we feel in an emergency, but still just as real.

Unresolved fear tends to keep the body under constant tension. Some people express this fear through their stomach as an ulcer; others express it through the colon as colitis. Still others have it show up in the lungs as asthma. Some express it through high blood pressure.

The octopus of anger and its internal tentacles of resentment, hatred, hostility, and bitterness have negative chemistry effects. All of these negative feelings tend to elevate our blood pressure. If you have a hypertension problem, go back and review the "chemistry of negative feelings" and the "healing of memories" (chapters 11 and 12). I'm not saying all essential hypertension is due to unresolved fear and anger, but I believe a significant amount is.

The tests we do to evaluate hypertension are not totally sensitive or accurate 100 percent of the time. Your disease may not yet have reached the stage where it is detectable by means other than your blood pressure. But high blood pressure, regardless of its causes, is a destructive process; it must be treated to forestall its pathologic consequences. Treatment, in my opinion, should include the standard medications, nutritional therapy, and healing of your memories of past inner hurts.

Dealing With Hypertension Nutritionally

The first level of treating hypertension is *dieting and nutritional therapy.* There is considerable evidence that diet alone is sufficient in many cases.

Second, avoid salt! Salt must be excreted through the kidneys. Excessive salt intake tends to increase high blood pressure. Many people can control their blood pressure by limiting their salt intake.

Third, increase your intake of fluids, primarily water. The ideal fluid intake for the average person is eight eight-ounce glasses of fluid a day. At least four of those eight glasses should be water.

Fourth, obesity is often interrelated with high blood pressure, so *treating the overweight problems is a must as well.* Follow the basic concepts in chapter 14 about losing weight and the basic dietary recommendations in chapter 18.

Fifth, most hypertensive patients will need a mild diuretic or some other drug to control their blood pressure, at least at the onset.

One other note: large dosages of vitamin E may have an adverse effect on hypertension, as well as on heart disease.

20
Arthritis

There are millions of people in the world who suffer from arthritis—some statistics indicate as many as 30 million in the United States alone. It affects the young and the old alike.

The standard treatment offered by the medical profession is the "drugs only" approach. These medications act to reduce inflammation and swelling and to relieve pain and stiffness. This treatment deals primarily with the symptoms. Although somewhat retardant to the disease, the "drugs only" approach does little to bring about true remission and/or healing of the degenerative process.

The side effects of these drugs are sometimes as bad as or worse than the disease itself. However, I must say, they do provide tremendous relief from pain and suffering for many people, but drugs are *not* the only approach to this disabling malady. I have had many arthritis patients who have been significantly helped through nutrition.

Understanding the Dis—ease and the Disease

Arthritis is an inflammatory, degenerative disorder of the musculo-skeletal system—primarily the joints. A musculo-skeletal joint is made up of bone, connective tissue, cartilage, joint fluid, tendons, ligaments, blood vessels, lymph vessels, and nerves. A knee isn't just a knee; it is a very complex structural and functional system, primarily mechanical in nature.

There are basically two types of arthritis. One is excessive wear, causing the degeneration of a joint. Second is an inflammatory process, affecting all the joint tissues. Many times I find people confuse inflammation and infection. An inflammation is a toxic swelling reaction within a tissue—like a bruise or a mosquito bite. An infection is an inflammation caused by bacteria, a virus, or some kind of organism that invades and infects the tissues, such as a boil, polio, pneumonia, and so forth.

When you have an infection, you also have an inflammation. But when you have an inflammation, you don't necessarily have an infection. Arthritis is an inflammatory process. Only occasionally is it an infectious process as well. Rheumatoid and gouty arthritis are examples of a purely inflammatory type of arthritis.

These diseases are caused by toxic substances from outside the joint (such as the bloodstream) which cause an inflammation of the joint tissues. Invasion by a bacteria, such as TB (tuberculosis) or gonorrhea are infectious arthritic processes.

Osteoarthritis, on the other hand, is the degenerative and destructive wearing out of a joint. It's caused by too much use, injury, and/or a mechanical-structural imbalance. It can be caused by: one, the wearing out that comes with old age; two, a short leg problem in which one leg is two inches shorter than the other; and three, an injury such as a fracture, especially one that involved the internal surface of a joint.

For these structural problems, a good osteopath or an M.D. orthopedist, who specializes in manipulative therapy will probably be the most help. An injection technique known as prolo-therapy or sclero-therapy is often helpful in injury or degenerative problems. For the Prolo-therapy Association, write to Gustav A. Hemovall, M.D., 715 Lake St., Oak Park, Illinois 60301. For the Sclero-therapy Association, get in touch with J. D. ZeBranek, D.O., 7139 Merriman Road, Garden City, Michigan 48135.

The Importance of Diet

In my experience, both the degenerative and the inflammatory processes involve the nutrition of the patient. Poor nutrition tends to hasten the wearing-out process. It also predisposes the body's immune system to malfunction. It allows the toxic substances of gout and rheumatoid arthritis to more rapidly advance in their destructive processes.

In my experience, a special arthritic diet has proven to be very helpful. Patients who are helped the most are those who were hurting most and were willing to stick rigidly to the dieting regimen.

Not only do I change a person's diet, I also recommend a number of supplements. These all come from natural sources, such as herbs and grasses. The supplements I use are products produced by the Standard Process Company Labs, Inc., Milwaukee, Wisconsin 53201. Although the company does not sell retail, they will be able to direct you to a local supplier.

Spiritual Side of Arthritis

There is one other factor in this disease. Dr. Loring T. Swaim, a noted rheumatologist from Boston and Harvard Medical School, wrote the book *Arthritis, Medicine, and the Spiritual Law.* His basic concept is that the rheumatoid-arthritis problem often has its source in (or is acutely aggravated by) negative attitudes. He gives many examples of individuals whose arthritis was in good control or remission, until something happened to them, and they reacted in a negative, hostile manner. At that point they had a tremendous flare-up of arthritic pain, swelling, and stiffness.

Often a rheumatoid-arthritic patient is a pleasant kindly person on the outside but inside he has a deep bitterness and hostility over some bad experience. There is usually also bitterness toward God "for letting this happen to me."

When we deal with negative feelings such as this, it is very difficult to be honest with ourselves about our true feelings. This is particularly true if we've been brought up in an environment in which the expression of anger is taboo; we have been impressed with the false ideal that any person who expresses such feelings is unacceptable and/or unchristian. But, in suppressing these feelings, we create physical disease for ourselves. If you have rheumatoid arthritis, I encourage you to read again chapters 10 to 13, and let God help you apply His principles discussed there.

The Seven-Day Diet

This nutritional program begins with a week-long general cleansing and detoxification regimen. It is particularly aimed at lower-bowel cleansing. You must reverse the process of the disease caused by poor diet. You must rid yourself of the effects of self-pollution that are the result of your mistakes in living. I realize, as you must, that this diet is not going to be easy. It will take a strong decision in favor of health. Once made—and stuck with—it will bring about a wonderful cleansing in the body. See how creative you can be with the foods given you. In this Seven-Day regimen, all of your body systems will tend to return to a more healthy state. Some people notice a significant improvement in this period of time, for others it takes thirty to sixty days.

Night before Day 1—Take mild laxative of your choice.
DAY 1—BREAKFAST Prune juice, banana.
         LUNCH All the raw vegetables you want.
         3:00 P.M. 2 glasses of water or diluted juice.
         6:00 P.M. 2 glasses of water or diluted juice.
         9:00 P.M. water or diluted juice as desired.
DAY 2—BREAKFAST 2 glasses water or diluted juice.
         10:00 A.M. 2 glasses of water or diluted juice.
         LUNCH 2 glasses of water or diluted juice.
         2:30 P.M. 2 glasses of water or diluted juice.
         Every meal raw vegetables.
         SNACKS Raw fresh fruit (no citrus).
DAY 3—BREAKFAST Raw fruits. Tomato juice (or
         tomato-vegetable juice mix). Nuts (such as a few almonds
         or walnuts).
         LUNCH Fresh fish. Raw fresh vegetables. Nuts (such as
         pecans or hickory nuts).
         DINNER Liver with onions, cole slaw or mixed-
         green salad, vegetable juice (tomato, celery,
         carrot, and so forth).
DAY 4—BREAKFAST Prunes, or prune juice, raw
         certified milk (if you can find it. No substitutes!).
         Nuts (be moderate).
         LUNCH Fresh organ meat (liver, kidney, heart,
         and so forth), green salad (use raw vegetables), vegetable

juice, small glass of raw certified milk.
DINNER Fresh seafood, raw fresh vegetables,
half an avocado (put oil and vinegar on it), and
nuts (hazel nuts and cashews).

DAY 5—BREAKFAST Fresh fruit (a good melon or
strawberries—no citrus!), nuts, raw certified
milk.
LUNCH Salad (avocado, tomato, spinach,
mushroom), raw certified milk.
DINNER Liver (this is important to cleasing),
fresh salad, fruit in season, vegetable juice,
olives.

DAY 6—BREAKFAST Prunes or prune juice, kidney
cooked lightly, nuts, raw certified milk.
LUNCH Fresh fish, raw fruit salad.
DINNER Hefty salad (lightly steamed or stir-
fried peas and string beans are great!), greens
(learn to grow your own sprouts), nuts, raw
certified milk.

DAY 7—BREAKFAST Bananas and raisins with
molasses, raw certified milk.
LUNCH Fresh fish, raw vegetables (cucumbers
and celery are excellent), fresh fruit, raw certified
milk.
DINNER Organ meat or fresh ocean fish,
vegetable juice (with a juicer you can mix a
number of juices together), raw fruit salad, raw
certified milk.

One tablespoon of molasses (unsulphured) per day will provide
minerals, a healthful sweetener, and also a laxative effect. Nutritional supplements which should be added:
3 Diaplex (Formula 17606) before each meal, 1
bottle, 7 days.
2 Comfrey-Pepsin E-3 after each meal, 1 bottle
(large), use all.
3 Senaplex (Formula 37806) after each meal, 1
bottle, 7 days.
(Prepared by the Standard Process Company Labs, Inc.)

Your New Diet

Once you have completed the Seven-Day cleaning-out period, you are ready to begin a twelve-week regimen. Continue your diet by avoiding refined carbohydrates. As we have said before, avidly avoid sugar, syrups (except pure maple, molasses, and honey). Also do not eat wheat (flour, cereals, and so forth), milk and milk products (except raw certified milk and cheese), deep-fat fried foods, and citrus. Some arthritis patients find that avoiding foods of the nightshade class (the family "solanaceous") helps to reduce their symptoms. They are: eggplant, potatoes, tomatoes, peppers, jalopeno, chili peppers, ground cherry, and red peppers.

Except for those food items you are not to eat, go over the lists of possible fruits, vegetables, and seafoods found in chapter 5 and add as much variety to your diet as possible. Make healthful living your hobby. Keep abreast of the latest scientific developments that affect food and water. Make certain you have a good cleaning out bowel movement every day. Keep looking for new and healthier ways to prepare food so it is appealing and delicious.

Take the following dietary supplements (also produced by Standard Process Company Labs):

2 Zypan before each meal; 2 bottles per month.
2 Rumaplex (Formula 3359 Plus) after each meal; 1 large bottle per 25 days.
1 Ostarplex (Formula 22159) after each meal; 1 bottle per 26 days.
1 Protefood with lunch; 1 bottle per 25 days.
2 Comfrey-Pepsin E-3 after each meal. Use remainder from first week of diet.

At the end of the twelve-week arthritic diet regimen, evaluate yourself. See how you feel, compared to before you started. How's your energy level now, as compared to what it was before? Are your joints as stiff and swollen? Do you have as much pain and discomfort? Estimate your overall improvement on a scale of "ten to zero." "Ten" is feeling well and good; "zero" is feeling miserable. If you have improved significantly, that should be good motivation to keep up this food plan and maintain what you've gained.

This is a continuing program. The supplements and the diet should be continued, if you want to keep the improvements you

have gained. Good health takes work and you must stay motivated
to keep on a good diet.

21

Constipation and/or Chronic Diarrhea

"Oh, I've been constipated all my life. But sometimes I have diarrhea for a day or two as well." This is a common complaint I receive from patients.

It is generally accepted in preventive Wholistic Medicine that it
is normal to have at least one good "cleaning-out" bowel movement a day. Many people have two.

When I ask other patients if they are constipated, they usually
reply, "Oh, no." But when I ask if they skip days, they will often
reply, "Oh, yes, I skip a day or two every week." That's what they
are used to, but that is not necessarily normal. Others say, "I skip
three or four days, then I have diarrhea for a day." This, of course,
is quite abnormal. One of my patients stated she had once gone
three weeks without a bowel movement.

On the other hand, I have patients with chronic diarrhea who
have ten or twelve diarrhea movements a day. One patient, after
she had corrected her diet and I placed her on the proper supplements, was quite pleased to find the number of her daily bowel
movements was reduced from ten to three or four.

Both constipation and non-infectious diarrhea are civilized diseases. They are the result of changes from a natural, rural life-style
to an urban inactive "civilized" approach to diet and life.

Dr. Denis Burkitt, a medical missionary to Africa, was an astute
investigator of the role of bulk and fiber in the diet. He observed
that native Africans in their tribal environment suffered little, if
any, stomach or bowel problems. Seldom did they have constipation, appendicitis, gallstones, colitis, colon cancer, or other gastro-

intestinal bowel diseases. However, those that moved to the city, in fifteen or twenty years, began to have these diseases.

Through some ingenious studies, Dr. Denis Burkitt found that the transit time (the time from eating to elimination) was significantly longer in those on the civilized diets than those on the native diet. The average transit time for a native was eighteen to thirty hours. For the city dweller, it ranged from two to seven days. The essential difference in the two diets was the amount of fiber and bulk.

The native diet was largely natural, unprocessed fruits and vegetables. Thus, the tribal natives were eating only high bulk and fiber and unrefined complex carbohydrate foods. The diet of the city dwellers was just the opposite.

The treatment of both constipation and chronic diarrhea is very much the same in some respects, quite different in others. Both require a diet high in bulk, fiber, or mucins. In diarrhea the bulk should be soft and fine. Coarse, heavy bulk such as celery, lettuce, and carrots, especially if not chewed well, may be too harsh to start with. Wheat bran, run through the blender and soaked, as well as fibrous fresh vegetables, chopped fine or blended, would be good for both. Also, drink lots of liquid.

With both of these problems, there is a malnutrition of the gastrointestinal bowel lining. I have found that dehydrated stomach, intestinal, and pancreatic tissue have a healing effect. These substances come in either powder or tablet form. With both constipation and diarrhea, the patient often needs the standard medical treatment, as well as nutritional supplements.

Chronic constipation, especially of long duration, responds best to a bowel-conditioning regimen. In addition to increasing the usual bulk, fluids, and nutrients, it is often advantageous to begin with a juice fast and a bowel conditioner. The one to use should contain the general ingredients of psyllium seed (both powder and husks of psyllium seed), papain, gum Karaya, sweet whey, fruit pectin, and prune powder. I recommend Mucovata, a bowel conditioner produced by Seroyal Brands, Inc., Concord, California 94524. It may require using this reconditioner one to two weeks to nudge the patient back into a normal bowel-evacuation pattern.

A good cleaning-out bowel movement every day is important. A delay in the transit time of any food containing a carcinogen (cancer-causing chemical) allows the cancer-causing chemical to be in contact with the lining of the bowel for a longer period of time. The longer the contact, the greater the possibility a cancer will begin. Also, the liver excretes cholesterol in the bile, which is emptied into the small intestine. Cholesterol is reabsorbed from the large bowel back into the body. A long transit time allows for greater reabsorption. A short transit time means less reabsorption of the cholesterol. (*See* chapter 18, on "Strokes and Hardening of the Arteries.")

In chronic diarrhea I often prescribe an inert, absorbent type of clay called bentonite. A little of this over a long period is better than a large amount all at once. Because it is an absorbing substance, overuse could cause mineral imbalance.

22
Colds and "The Flu"

There really isn't a flu season anymore; there are simply times when the Hong Kong or the Asian flu pass through.

Each kind of flu is just a different strain of virus causing the same symptoms and/or disease. Our bodies are able to overcome most viral infections without the use of antibiotics or other drug medications. However, when a viral infection breaks down the body's resistance sufficiently, we are very susceptible to secondary bacterial infections, such as tonsillitis or pneumonia and so on.

Treatment of Colds and Flu

For the initial stages of treating a cold or the flu, I find the first thing to do is to *rest*. If you are starting to come down with the flu, but compulsively go to work, you are doing yourself and your associates a great disfavor. The first twenty-four to forty-eight hours of any flu or cold are usually the worst and the most contagious. Besides being inefficient, you will be passing on your flu or cold to everyone with whom you come into contact. Just one cough in an elevator or office is enough to spread those viral particles to every-one within ten to fifteen feet. So stay home and get lots of rest.

Second, you will want to *force fluids.* Fix yourself a pitcher of warm lemonade or diluted fruit juice. Drink four or five eight-ounce glasses (for adults), over a period of an hour. Doing this once or twice a day tends to trip the diuretic mechanism. You will then rapidly flush off through your kidneys the toxic products, which are the result of your illness. Getting these toxic elements out of your system as quickly as possible helps you feel better faster.

Warm liquids tend to have an internal soothing effect; they pro-mote circulation, and help relieve the chills. Drinking four or five glasses of ice-cold liquid would have a negative effect. It would cause chilling, which tends to stimulate the production of more histamine and increases the symptoms of the flu or cold.

When you're nauseated and are vomiting, drink a warm, con-centrated, salt solution in the form of a broth or bouillon. For an adult, one-half teaspoon of salt in half a cup of water is enough. Sip it down slowly. Concentrated salt water tends to have a cleansing effect on the stomach. If you have been vomiting, the salts in the bouillon will help replace the salt and other minerals you have lost. Vomiting and diarrhea are the main ways you lose salt from the body, although profuse sweating will also deplete your electrolyte minerals.

The Importance of Vitamin C

Third, I am convinced most viral problems can be greatly helped by *taking adequate amounts of vitamin C.* Start by taking at least one gram every hour. When you have reached your tolerance of vitamin C for the day, you develop a loose stool or a small amount of diarrhea. Stop taking vitamin C and begin again the next day with a lesser amount. People with colds or flu can tolerate upwards to fifteen or forty grams or more of vitamin C a day.

I attended an International Academy of Applied Nutrition con-ference a few years ago. One of the doctors gave a well-docu-mented presentation on treating viral pneumonia with vitamin C. In treating one patient, he gave 210 milligrams of vitamin C both orally and through IVs the first day. The second day, he gave the patient 180 mgs.; the third day, 160 mgs. By the end of one week's period, as evidenced by the X rays, the patient had completely resolved the pneumonia process. The doctor had also used customary antibiotics. However, the patient recovered at an exceptionally fast rate—much faster than normally expected.

Vitamin C has a second advantage. If you take enough, it tends to clean out your bowel. If you are constipated, and stay that way for two or three days, it is more difficult for the body to rid itself of toxic substances that are the result of the cold or flu.

Although it is important to clean out the bowels during a cold or the flu, it would not be a good idea to take a harsh laxative during such a disease process. Though it would clean the bowel, it also tends to create mineral electrolyte and vitamin deficiencies in the body.

A good substitute for aspirin is calcium lactate. Taking these tablets on an empty stomach tends to be fever relieving. An adult can take fifteen to twenty tablets a day for a fever over 102 degrees. It should be noted a temperature up to 101 degrees is not one to be overly concerned about. A slight temperature elevation indicates the body is reacting to the disease process with favorable results. It restricts the growth of the virus because they do not grow as well at 102 degrees. If your fever gets over 105 degrees it's important to treat it with a cooling regimen of an ice-water sponge bath, and aspirin, and a call to your doctor.

With a fever, particularly where there is an excessive amount of sweating, vomiting, and diarrhea, you need to be concerned about the loss of potassium. Often the feeling of fatigue and weakness that comes after a siege of severe sweating, vomiting, or diarrhea is due to a potassium depletion. This is especially true if you have been on water pills (diuretics). Taking a potassium supplement and eating foods with high potassium content may relieve that weak and washed-out feeling. Potassium should be used with great caution, however, especially in small children. Too much can be as bad as too little.

Summary:
The Good Chemistry of Peace of
Mind

I just talked to my editor, who said, "It's all done except for a summary chapter." So after four years and thousands of pages of writes and rewrites, I find myself again confronted with the questions "Why am I writing this book?" "What am I trying to say?"

I think both questions can be answered with the same answer: *nutrition!* It was the basic problem and answer for at least fifteen of the twenty patients I saw today. To me, nutrition is both what you feed your body and what you feed your soul.

My first patient started at 6:00 A.M. This forty-five-year-old man's first comment was, "I'm basically healthy; I just want to know how to eat right." However, he responded with many positive answers to the "Signs and Symptoms" questions as outlined in chapter 3.

Next was a phone call from an anxious husband. His wife has had a problem of gross obesity for many, many years. She has been halfheartedly on and off diets all of her adult life. Now she is beginning to show laboratory signs of multiple metabolic diseases: hypertension, gout, diabetes, liver disease, kidney disease, all of which have life-threatening implications. I had referred her to a specialty clinic for high-risk obesity patients. Their literature listed all of the major possible complications of treatment, one of which is death. Medical-legal factors now make it necessary to tell a patient all the possible serious side effects of a medical or surgical treatment. She had panicked at even the thought of that remote possibility. I tried to explain to him that the risk of not doing anything about her serious medical problem was greater than the risk of the therapy used by the specialty clinic. For her to go to Weight Watchers, Overeaters Anonymous, Tops, even with careful medical supervision, would be a definite risk. (In fact, getting out of bed in the morning is a risk. Driving the freeway to work is a risk. Taking aspirin is a risk.) I urged him to have her follow through, even though she was frightened of the possible complications.

Next was a nine-year-old with huge tonsils, eustachian-tube blockage, a hearing problem, multiple allergies and anemia—all basically physical nutritional problems.

Next was a sixty-five-year-old lady, depressed, anxious, nervous, tired, no energy, stomach pain, and lots of guilt feelings, because she wasn't able to keep up with all the things she felt she "had to do." Her guilt and fears had so overstressed her already-nutritionally deficient body, she was totally unable to cope. She had had thousands of dollars of tests and many hours of counseling before she was referred to me. No one had ever questioned her about her nutrition. Her diet diary was horrible.

Next was a three-year-old with a seizure problem. He does very well, that is, has no seizures, unless he eats something that has sugar in it. He has learned at that very young age he can avoid those terrifying seizures by not eating sweets. His mother stated that now when someone offers him a cookie or a sucker he says, "No, I can't eat that. It makes me sick."

Why so much nutritional disease in our Age of Scientific Advancement?

The big hang-up, as I see it, is our eating habits. From birth we begin eating what we are fed. Then we begin eating by taste and/or the gimmick advertising of the media. In my young days, it was Jack Armstrong and Little Orphan Annie; then television took over. We were programmed into our habits of eating with little or no awareness of what balanced, good nutrition is.

We learned to like and dislike on the basis of taste, texture, and eye appeal. What was quick, easy, and convenient was the ideal. We eat many different food entities or chemicals all in the same meal. We never stop to think about foods as chemicals that affect our ability to think and feel. After all, we've been eating these same foods all our lives. How could they be bad for us? I thought bread and cheese and steak were good for you—and potatoes and green beans! They may be, but none of these are perfect foods. They are all deficient in some of the essential nutrients. Eating the same depleted food over and over is the best way there is to develop food sensitivities and allergies.

It is also the best way to develop nutritional deficiencies of minerals and vitamins that are *essential* to proper functioning of our mind and emotions.

At least 75 percent of all the foods you eat, unless you are extremely careful, are deficient or missing entirely many of the nutrients they contained in the natural state.

The mistaken concept of "Oh, I thought that was good for you," is one I do battle with every day. Just yesterday a thirty-two-year-old-woman was back to see me for her three-week evaluation, after I had taken her completely off milk and wheat. "The first few days," she commented, "were terrible. I felt bad, had a headache, was mentally foggy and confused. I was so tired I could hardly do anything. But now I feel better than I have in a long time. My head is clear and I can think better. I have lots more energy. Even my face is much clearer than it's been for a long time. I've known for a long, long time something was wrong. I guess one just grows into it so gradually, you don't really know the difference. You get to believing not feeling good is normal.

"I've always tried to eat right. I read all the time about preventive medicine and nutrition. I'm sure that I was eating wheat and milk products before I can even remember. Probably since birth. I just never stopped to think that they might be what was making me feel bad all the time."

Our Physical Comes First

In Genesis we find our origin, our roots, come from the dust of the ground. God created man, first, a chemical being, then a living soul. We were not first a spirit flitting around in space waiting for a body to be conceived!

Our physical body is the structural basis for our functions. "To feel" and "to know" are man's basic functions. Intellect isn't something separate from the body. Emotions, feelings, moods, nerves are all a part of our body chemistry. Depression, anxiety, irritability, anger, bitterness, resentment are all negative chemistry. Love, hope, companionship, acceptance, being needed are positive chemistry.

The mind- and mood-altering effect of marijuana, heroin, cocaine, LSD, alcohol, aspirin, tranquilizers, antidepressants are all very well known. It is easy to accept that these are chemicals

which affect our ability "to know" and "to feel" and "to act."
But its almost unbelievable to most people that a food such as
milk, or wheat, or beef, or peanut butter would have a similar effect.

Deficiency, Sooner or Later, Means Disease

Energy is the final end point in the metabolism of all living
things. Without a constant optimum-energy flow there is no optimum life. Every chemical reaction in the human body—and there
are thousands of them in every cell—has something to do with energy. This energy flow is altered either by too much or too little of
the basic nutrients, or by toxic foreign substances. Yes, your body
can malfunction from having too much oxygen, water, or any of the
other essential nutrients, just as you do from having too little. An
optimum-energy level is dependent on optimum nutrition.

The most common complaint I hear is, "I just don't have enough
energy." "I have to push myself all the time. I can't get done all the
things I have to do."

All the symptoms listed in Chapter 3 (depression, anxiety, irritability, palpitations, light-headedness, and so forth) are related to a
lack of energy.

At least 90 percent of the patients who come to me for nutritional evaluation state they just don't have enough energy—they
are *tired.* Within one month after I've changed their diet and recommended a therapeutic supplement regimen, most of them say, "I
really feel so much better. I don't feel as tired as I used to. I really
didn't realize how bad I felt."

Learn to Listen to Your Body

It is the best measuring device you will ever have. Every feeling
you have—pain or pleasure—is the result of chemistry. It isn't evil
elves or witches or demons with pitchforks. Your feelings are your
body telling you what is right or what is wrong with it.

Stress—either good or bad—whether it's primarily physical or
completely mental and emotional has its end point in the body
mechanism. All stresses, regardless of their origin, have a physical
effect. You cannot express your mental-emotional self unless you
do it through your physical body. Love, tenderness, caring, em-

pathy, fear, anger, bitterness, resentment, or whatever feeling you are feeling are all expressed through body chemistry. Your voice is a physical apparatus and it expresses your feelings. With your eyes you can look loving or look hating. You can touch tenderly or give a blow in anger. All are feelings expressed as chemical reactions through your physical mechanism. The greater the stress, the more energy it takes to cope, and the faster we burn up our nutrients to provide the energy we expend.

The last questions I ask each new patient are related to their own self-evaluation and their ability to cope with stress.

Are you a happy person?

What do you do for fun?

When was your last resting get-away vacation of at least two weeks?

What was your biggest disappointment and/or your deepest hurt?

Answers to the first three tell me how highly you value yourself and how well you take care of you.

Your unresolved biggest disappointment and/or deepest hurt tells me of your energy drains.

Most people can almost instantly replay some experience that has deeply and negatively affected their lives. Almost without exception, there is a deep, deep sense of having been wronged—a sense of personal injustice. This sense of having been wronged and/or of personal injustice stimulates a very negative chemistry in the body. It's the catecholamine-adrenalin chemistry of fear and flight or fight—the chemistry of anger, bitterness, revenge, hatred, loneliness, despair, and hopelessness. These are the greatest energy drainers there are.

There is a great amount of clinical evidence that such negative "stress reactions" play a critical role in the release of most disease processes within the body. Cancer, arthritis, heart attacks, ulcers, colitis are but a few. Voodoo death, that is, by the placing of a hex on a person, is probably the most dramatic example. On the other hand, when one is happy, joyful, filled with hope and can be thankful in whatever circumstance one finds oneself, one promotes very positive healing, renewing chemistry within the body. These emotions stimulate the production of endorphins, the healing, stress-releasing chemicals of the brain and nervous system.

"But how can anyone be happy and grateful for a wrong and/or an injustice?" you ask. Simple. Without an injustice we would have been denied the greatest joy man can experience, that is salvation. If Jesus had been treated justly, He never would have been crucified. Right? Right! Without Jesus' having been crucified, there would have been no shedding of blood for the forgiveness of sin.

Without having been Victim of the cross, Jesus could never have become *Victor* over the cross and death and hell. There would have been no Resurrection on Easter morning. So rejoice and be grateful for an injustice. There is no wrong, no injustice that Jesus is not able to become Victor over. How many times have I heard my friend and patient Corrie ten Boom say, "Jesus is VICTOR." Certainly she and her family experienced a terrible injustice, but through that injustice, God was able to show His love to millions of people in hundreds of countries around the world.

You, too, can find hope and happiness and peace of mind.

1   Confess you have failed to love enough. Sin is failing to love enough.
2   Ask God to reveal Himself to you. Knowledge of God comes only through revelation (Matthew 16:17).
3   Receive Him. "Behold, I stand at the door and knock; if any one hears My voice and opens the door, I will come in to him . . . (Revelation 3:20).
4   Know that you have everlasting life. "These things I have written to you who believe in the name of the Son of God, in order that you may know that you have eternal life" (1 John 5:13).

It sounds too simple, doesn't it? It is; it's so simple it's the most difficult choice any of us will ever make. But it's worth it.

Release the grudges, the bitterness, the wish for vengeance that you are clutching so dearly to your breast. Let them go. Free yourself from these negative emotions that create disease. Then listen to your body. Let it tell you as much as it can. Eat wisely, and you will have the best of good health and happiness and peace of mind that it is possible to have!

Appendixes

Appendix A
The Diet Diary

RC Refined carbohydrates are usually the chief ingredients of junk foods. They are characterized by prepreparation, refining, processing, and purifying or chemical texturizing, coloring, preserving, and stabilizing. Not included in this category are those which are involved in cooking, canning, freezing, aging, pickling, or fermenting (as in sauerkraut).

Refined Carbohydrate List

1 All sugars are refined: white, brown, raw, maple, tupelo, and so forth
2 White "wheat" flour, enriched or bleached or unbleached
3 Cornstarch
4 Sugar-based gelatins
5 Peeled potatoes, fried, French fried, mashed, scalloped, hashed browns, and so forth
6 White rice
7 Highly refined and processed prepared cereals, dry or quick-cooked

M Milk and milk products are desirable for most people but are not necessary for a balanced diet. These include such milk products as milk cheese, cottage cheese, yogurt, ice cream, powdered milk, custards, and so forth. It does not, however, include such dairy products as butter and eggs.

W Wheat includes white or wheat flour (bleached or unbleached, enriched or not) and wheat germ, as well as the whole-wheat products. (If you are allergic to wheat, it doesn't matter whether it is refined or whole.) You should include *all* wheat-containing foods in your Diet Diary.

F and O Fats and oils include not only such products as butter and salad oil, but also foods prepared in deep fat. Consider also margarines, shortening, lard, and oil-based dressings (such as Roquefort, Thousand Island), and dips for chips.

F and M Fruits and melons are easily identified. Do *not* include commercially prepared ones with sugar.

183

   V **Vegetables** vary in food value according to their preparation. Six servings a day are recommended, at least half to be eaten raw.

Stim **Stimulants,** such as coffee, tea, cola, and alcohol should be recorded carefully.

   P **Proteins** are most commonly found in meats, poultry, fish, shellfish, and also found in eggs, milk products, and vegetable proteins.

As indicated on the following sample charts, some foods will fall into more than one category. My analysis of a patient's eating habits through the use of these Diet Diaries can uncover unbalanced diets and might even provide significant clues to food allergies or sensitivity responses.

"Quiet Times" are times you stop what you are doing and just do nothing—relax—meditate—cut yourself off from the world for a few moments to renew your inner self.

(*See page 86 for instructions on taking your pulse.*)

Sample diet diary forms follow.

Diet Diary For: _John DOE_

Starting Date: _11-21-79_

Sex: _Male_ Age: _62_

Day of Week: 1			Arising Temp. 97.1	Arising Pulse: 62
How slept? Good	No. Quiet Times?		Moods, Feeling Level	Physical Problems (Headache, Cramps, Other)
Time of Day 8:30	Morning Meal ½ grapefruit / frosted flakes / coffee / sugar	FM / RC / Stim / RC	Depressed Hard to get up	Time of Day 6:30 am
	Snack	None	Light-headed	11:00 — Headache
1:00	Lunch soup / crackers / cheese / ice cream vanilla / cookies / iced tea	W / M / M RC / RC W / Stim	Tired Groggy Sleepy	2:30 — Headache Throbbing
	Snack			
6:30	Evening Meal soup / chicken chow mein / cookies / tea	P / RC W / Stim	Nausea	7:30 — Stomach cramps Diarrhea
11:00 pm	Snack after the Choc. pie show	RC		
	Type of Exercise Walking			Length of Time 30 min.

Diet Diary For: _John Doe_

Starting Date: _11-21-79_

Sex: _Male_ Age: _62_

Day of Week: 2		Arising Temp. 96.8		Arising Pulse: 62	
How slept? Good	No. Quiet Times?	Moods, Feeling Level		Physical Problems (Headache, Cramps, Other)	
Time of Day	Morning Meal				
8:00	frosted flakes — RC coffee — Stim sugar — RC	Tired Feel confused	Time of Day	Diarrhea 2am 6am	
		Anxious Tense Irritable	11:30		
	Snack				
1:30	Lunch				
	salad — V barbecued pork — P barbecued beans — V French fried potato — FO RC white bread — W RC iced tea — Stim	Dizzy Light-headed	2:30	Sense of bloating abnormal fullness, like food didn't digest well	
	Snack	Tired Exhausted Mind confused	5:30	Lots of gas	
8:00	Evening Meal				
	cheese sandwich — M butter — FO white bread — W coffee — Stim sugar — RC				
	Snack	Depressed Anxious		Constipated No BM today	
	Type of Exercise Walking			Length of Time 45 min.	

Diet Diary For: _John Doe_
Starting Date: _11-21-79_
Sex: _Male_ Age: _62_

Day of Week: 3		Arising Temp. 97.0		Arising Pulse: 58	
How slept? Good	No. Quiet Times?	Moods, Feeling Level		Physical Problems (Headache, Cramps, Other)	
Time of Day	Morning Meal		Time of Day	Headache
8:30	fried egg FO P white toast RC W butter FO coffee Stim sugar RC	Fairly good		
	Snack None	Irritable Grouchy Had a fight with the man next door		
2:00	Lunch salad V fried pork chop FO P canned peas V cranberries FM white bread RC W butter FO iced tea Stim	Feel wrung out Anxious Shaking a lot Cold sweats	3:00 pm	Bloated feeling again Too full but didn't eat that much
	Snack None		6:30 pm	Lots of gas
	Evening Meal None	Mind foggy Can't keep my attention on what I am doing		
8:00	Snack Mounds candy bar RC	Too tired To bed	8:00 pm	Constipated No BM
	Type of Exercise Walking			Length of Time 45 min.

Diet Diary For: _John Doe_

Starting Date: _11-21-79_

Sex: _Male_   Age: _62_

Day of Week: 4			Arising Temp. 97.0		Arising Pulse: 60
How slept? Good	No. Quiet Times?		Moods, Feeling Level		Physical Problems (Headache, Cramps, Other)
Time of Day	Morning Meal			Time of Day	
8:30	½ grapefruit French toast syrup butter coffee sugar	FM W RC FO Stim RC	Hard to get up Tense Irritable Feel blah No energy Washed out	1:00	Headache (severe)
					Light-headed Dizzy all day
	Snack				
					Nausea—from paint fumes
3:00	Lunch				
	T-bone steak barbequed cabbage salad sweet pickle white bread butter iced tea	P V V W RC FO Stim			
	Snack		Too tired Mind blurred Went to bed	5:30	
	Evening Meal	X			Constipated No BM—3rd day
			Restless Can't sleep	10:45	Took Ex-lax
	Snack glass milk crackers	M W	Tossing and turning		
10:45	Type of Exercise Painted bedroom 9:30–1:30				Length of Time 4 hours

Diet Diary For: _John Doe_
Starting Date: _11-21-79_
Sex: _Male_ Age: _62_

Day of Week: 5			Arising Temp. 97.2	Arising Pulse: 55	
How slept? Good	No. Quiet Times?		Moods, Feeling Level		Physical Problems (Headache, Cramps, Other)
Time of Day	Morning Meal			Time of Day	
8:30	fried egg bacon white toast jam coffee sugar	FO P FO RC W RC Stim RC	Tired Hard to get up	8:00 am	Headache (bad)
			Feeling like I'm going to faint	11:00 am	
	Snack		Rapid heartbeat Shakes		
1:30	Lunch		Severe sweating Anxious and nervous		
	stewed chicken noodles chicken gravy biscuits iced tea	P W RC W RC W Stim		3:00 pm	Heavy, bloated feeling in stomach like food hasn't digested well
			Exhausted Too tired to think		
4:00	Snack regular Dr. Pepper Stim RC			5:00 pm	
	Evening Meal				
				7:00	Diarrhea
				8:00	Diarrhea
				9:30	Diarrhea
8:30	Snack coffee Stim sugar RC orange FM				
	Type of Exercise Walking			Length of Time 45 min.	

Appendix B
Test Day Forms

Test Day Forms are a simple way to help you test yourself for a specific food allergy. Use them for any food that you feel might be causing you to react adversely. This test is best done in the morning because your digestive system will be comparatively free of food.

It is important to note any change in your mental, emotional, and physical feelings. What you feel is what's most important in this testing procedure. If you feel any of the symptoms listed on the form below (or others that are not listed), grade them on a scale of 0 to 4. Zero should be considered as normal; *1* is a slight feeling of discomfort; *2* is a moderate feeling of discomfort; *3* is a significant feeling of discomfort; and *4* would indicate marked or severe symptoms.

As an example of how to test foods, I have included samples of two specific foods: milk and wheat.

MILK (OR OTHER FOODS*) CHALLENGE OR TEST DAY

No other foods or drink except water and milk, cheese, or yogurt (*or other specified foods, such as peanut butter, oranges, soybeans, or eggs) can be eaten during the course of this test.

First, record your pulse and any symptoms.

Then drink two glasses of milk (nothing else).

At one hour after drinking the milk, record your pulse and any symptoms.

At the second hour, record your pulse and any symptoms. Then have your second serving of milk or milk products. You may drink milk or have a large serving of cheese or yogurt.

At the third hour, record your pulse and any symptoms.

Fourth hour, record your pulse and any symptoms.

It is important to note any change in your mental, emotional, and physical feelings. Remember, what you feel is what is important! After you have finished this food test, you may fast the rest of the day or resume your regular diet. IF YOU FEEL NO REACTION, REPEAT THE MILK TEST AS ABOVE A SECOND DAY.

If you feel any of the symptoms listed below, or others, grade them from 1+ to 4+.

1+ would be a slight feeling.
2+ would be a moderate feeling.
3+ would be significant or a lot.
4+ would be marked or severe symptoms.

Milk Test-Day Form

	Day 1 fasting	Day 1 1st milk challenge 1	Day 1 2	Day 1 2nd milk challenge 3	Day 1 4	Day 2 fasting	Day 2 1st milk challenge 1	Day 2 2	Day 2 2nd milk challenge 3	Day 2 4
TIME OF DAY										
PULSE										
Weakness										
Tremors										
Cold Sweat										
Palpitations										
Dizziness										
Anxiety										
Headache										
Tired										
Sleepy										
Nausea										
Stomach Aches/ Cramps										
Mental Confusion										
Fainting/Light-headed										
Depression										

SYMPTOMS

GRAIN ALLERGY CHALLENGE OR TEST DAY,
example WHEAT

No other foods or drink except water and wheat (or the specified grain) can be eaten during the course of this test.

First, record your pulse.

Then, have your first wheat challenge, preferably a whole-grain cereal. You may have a pat of butter on the cereal, but no other grain, milk, sugar, sweeteners, or salt are allowed.

At one hour, record your pulse and any change in your feelings or symptoms.

At the second hour, record your pulse and any symptoms. Then have your second wheat challenge.

At the third hour, record your pulse and any symptoms.

Fourth hour, record your pulse and any symptoms. Have your third serving of wheat.

At the fifth and sixth hours, record your pulse and any symptoms.

It is important to note any change in your mental, emotional, and physical feelings. Remember, what you feel is what is important! After you have finished this food test, you may fast the rest of the day, or resume your regular diet.

If you feel any of the symptoms listed below, or others, grade them from 1+ to 4+.

1+ would be a slight feeling.
2+ would be a moderate feeling.
3+ would be very significant or a lot.
4+ would be marked or severe symptoms.

Grain Test-Day Form

		fasting	1st food challenge		2nd food challenge		3rd food challenge					
			1	2	3	4	5	6				
TIME OF DAY												
PULSE												
SYMPTOMS	Weakness											
	Tremors											
	Cold Sweat											
	Palpitations											
	Dizziness											
	Anxiety											
	Headache											
	Tired											
	Sleepy											
	Nausea											
	Stomach Aches/ Cramps											
	Mental Confusion											
	Fainting/Light-headed											
	Depression											

Appendix C
Food Sensitivity Testing Forms

Test one food only every two hours.

Cereals: Test the grains only in three successive feedings, Wheatena or Roman Meal, oats, oatmeal (*For all other foods, one food-test challenge is enough.*)

Fruits: apple, grapes, banana, melon, orange, peach, pineapple, avocado, cantaloupe, grapefruit

Protein: beef, chicken, fish, pork, egg

Nuts and Seeds: almonds, peanuts, peanut butter

Vegetables: tomato, mushroom, cucumber, cabbage, potato, beets, sweet potato, string beans, corn, lettuce

Beverages: water, coffee, milk, soy milk, yeast drinks

Food Sensitivity Testing

Name _____

Date _____

Pulse Rate beats per minute before eating	Food	Time	Pulse Rate one hour after eating	Reaction or Responses

Appendix D
Glucose Tolerance Test Forms

The purpose of a five-hour glucose tolerance test (5hr GTT) is to identify the symptoms experienced by a patient when he/she is subjected to a refined carbohydrate overload.

I do not ask my patients to do a high-carbohydrate-loading diet before the test, since this is not their customary way of eating. I prefer to see how they respond to a high-carbohydrate challenge, just the way they would if they ate a hot-fudge sundae, or a piece of apple pie a la mode.

Each patient fills out a symptom check-sheet during the course of the test. How the patient reacts during the test is much more important than the change in milligram percentage values on a 5hr GTT graph.

On Graph A the numbers are not out of the normal range. However, the symptoms experienced by this patient during the course of the test are very positive. This patient's blood sugar level did not fall to 50 mg. or below, and so he could not be classified technically as being a hypoglycemic. However, the sugar itself, or a minute residual of some chemical used in processing the sugar, was present in sufficient quantity to create adverse symptoms.

How the patient feels is most important. The numbers are important only if they are persistently high, as on Graph B, or if there is a rapid drop to the *low 50* range accompanied by marked symptoms as illustrated in Graph C.

My five-hour glucose tolerance test includes taking an extra blood specimen at three and one-half hours, which is very seldom included in the standard test routine.

It is my experience that 10 percent or more of glucose tolerance tests will show a positive curve by including a three-and-a-half hour specimen.

This is clearly illustrated in Graph C. The standard test taken only at three and four hours would not have shown a positive test for hypoglycemia.

Glucose Tolerance Test-A

Name _____

Date _____

Sex _____

Age _____

Please leave this form with the Lab Technician when test is completed.

You should obtain a urine specimen 5 minutes before each of the following blood sample times: 10:35, 11:30, 12:00, 1:00, 2:00, 2:30, 3:00, 4:00.

If you should feel any of the following symptoms, grade the appropriate column from 1+ to 4+, 4+ being the worst.

	F	½	1	1½	2	2½	3	3½	4	4½	5
TIME OF DAY:											
Mg.% drop / Hyperglycemia — 400, 350, 300, 280, 260, 240, 220, 200, 190, 180, 170, 160, 150, 140, 130, 120			178			136					
Normal Range — 110, 105, 100, 95, 90, 85, 80, 75, 70	81						100			87	
Hypoglycemia — 65, 60, 55, 50, 45, 40, 35								71	65		
Blood sugar %											
Urine sugar %											

SYMPTOMS

	F	½	1	1½	2	2½	3	3½	4	4½	5
Weakness				1+	2+	2+	2+	2+	2+	2+	
Tremors					1+	1+	1+		1+	2+	
Cold Sweat					1+						
Palpitations											
Dizziness						1+	2+	2+	1+	1+	
Anxiety											
Headache											
Tired			1+			2+	2+	2+	2+	1+	
Sleepy											
Nausea	1+					1+	1+				
Stomach Aches/ Cramps											
Mental Confusion						1+	2+	1+	1+		
Fainting/Lt. headed											
Depression								1+			

Glucose Tolerance Test-B

Name _____

Date _____

Sex _____

Age _____

Please leave this form with the Lab Technician when test is completed.

You should obtain a urine specimen 5 minutes before each of the following blood sample times: 10:35, 11:30, 12:00, 1:00, 2:00, 2:30, 3:00, 4:00.

If you should feel any of the following symptoms, grade the appropriate column from 1+ to 4+, 4+ being the worst.

	F	½	1	1½	2	2½	3	3½	4	4½	5
TIME OF DAY:											

Mg.% drop

Hyperglycemia: 400 350 300 280 260 240 220 200 190 180 170 160 150 140 130 120

Normal Range: 110 105 100 95 90 85 80 75 70

Hypoglycemia: 65 60 55 50 45 40 35

(plotted values: 144, 203, 254, 320, 295, 265, 256, 177)

	F	½	1	1½	2	2½	3	3½	4	4½	5
Glucose	—	—	/+		4+		4+	4+	2+		—
Acetone	—	—	—		—		—	—	—		—

SYMPTOMS

Weakness											
Tremors											
Cold Sweat											
Palpitations											
Dizziness											
Anxiety											
Headache											
Tired											
Sleepy											
Nausea											
Stomach Aches/Cramps											
Mental Confusion											
Fainting/Lt. headed											
Depression											

Glucose Tolerance Test-C

Name _____

Date _____

Sex _____

Age _____

Please leave this form with the Lab Technician when test is completed.

You should obtain a urine specimen 5 minutes before each of the following blood sample times: 10:35, 11:30, 12:00, 1:00, 2:00, 2:30, 3:00, 4:00.

If you should feel any of the following symptoms, grade the appropriate column from 1+ to 4+, 4+ being the worst.

	F	½	1	1½	2	2½	3	3½	4	4½	5
TIME OF DAY:											
Blood sugar %											
Urine sugar %											
Weakness									/		/
Tremors									4		
Cold Sweat									4	2	/
Palpitations			/						/		
Dizziness											/
Anxiety		2+	2+	2+	3	2	2	1½	2	/	/
Headache		3+	/	2+	3				3	2	4
Tired		2	2	2	3	/		/			
Sleepy				2	2						
Nausea		/+	2	2	2				3	/	/
Stomach Aches/Cramps											
Mental Confusion		2+	2+	2	2+	/	/	/	/	/	/
Fainting/Lt. headed											
Depression											
Feel Feverish		/+	/+	/	/+	/	/	/	ColD	ColD	ColD
Neckache Eyes-Burn/Hurt		4/3+	4/3+	4/3	4/3	4/3	4/2+	4/1	4/1	4/1	4/1
Tense/Nervous		3	3	3	3	3	2	2	2	2	2

Suggested Reading

Suggested Reading

Natural Food Cookbooks

Albright, Nancy. *The Rodale Cookbook.* Emmaus, PA: Rodale Press, 1973.

Berto, Hazel. *Cooking With Honey.* New York: Gramercy Publishing Company, 1972.

Bragg, Paul C. and Patricia. *Hi-Protein, Meatless Health Recipes.* Santa Barbara, CA: Health Science, 1979.

Brooks, Karen, *The Forget-About-Meat Cookbook.* Emmaus, PA: From Arrowhead Mills. Rodale Press, 1974.

Ford, Frank. *The Simpler Life Cookbook.* Fort Worth: Harvest Press, 1978.

Hunter, Beatrice Trum. *Fact-Book on Fermented Foods and Beverages: An Old Tradition.* New Canaan, CT: Keats Publishing, 1973.

Rohrer, Norman and Virginia. *How to Eat Right and Feel Great.* Wheaton, IL: Tyndale House Publishers, 1977.

Smetinoff, Olga. *The Yogurt Cookbook.* New York: Pyramid Books, 1966.

Toms, Agnes. *The Joy of Eating Natural Foods.* Old Greenwich, CT: The Devin-Adair Company, 1962.

Natural Gardening Books

Cruso, Thalassa. *Making Vegetables Grow.* New York: Alfred A. Knopf, 1975.

Mabe, Rex E. *Gardening With Herbs.* Greensboro, NC: Potpourri Press, 1973.

Oliver, Martha H. *Add a Few Sprouts.* New Canaan, CT.: Keats Publishing, 1975.

Books on Physical Conditioning

Morehouse, Laurence E., and Gross, Leonard. *Total Fitness in Thirty Minutes a Week.* New York: Pocket Books, 1975.

Stern, Jess. *Dr. Thompson's New Way for You to Care for Your Aching Back.* New York: Doubleday & Co., Inc., 1979.

Van Aaken, Ernst. Translated by George Beinhorn. *Van Aaken Method: Finding the Endurance to Run Faster and Live Healthier.* Mountain View, CA: World Publications, 1976.

Books for Emotional-Spiritual Good Health

Becker, Ernest. *Escape From Evil.* New York: The Free Press, 1975.
Linn, Dennis and Linn, Matthew. *Healing Life's Hurts.* New York: Paulist Press, 1978.
Pfeiffer, Carl C., *et al. The Schizophrenias: Yours and Mine.* New York: Pyramid Books, 1970.
Schuller, Robert H. *Self-Love: The Dynamic Force of Success.* Old Tappan, NJ: Spire Books, 1969.
————*Turning Your Stress Into Strength.* Irvine, CA: Harvest House Publishers, 1978.
Trobisch, Walter. *Love Yourself.* Downers Grove, IL: Inter-Varsity Press, 1976.

Books on Nutrition

Adams, Ruth, and Frank Murray. *Minerals: Kill or Cure?* New York: Larchmont Books, 1974.
Brennan, R. O. *Nutrigenetics: New Concepts for Relieving Hypoglycemia.* New York: New American Library, 1977.
Elwood, Catharyn. *Feel Like a Million!* New York: Pocket Books, 1952.
Hall, Ross Hume. *Food for Nought: The Decline in Nutrition.* New York: Harper & Row, Publishers, 1974.
Kirschman, John D. *Nutrition Almanac.* New York: McGraw-Hill Book Company, 1973.
Kutsky, Roman J. *Handbook of Vitamins and Hormones.* New York: Van Nostrand Reinhold Company, 1973.
Newbold, H. L. *Mega-Nutrients for Your Nerves.* New York: Wyden Books, 1975.
Pfeiffer, Carl C., *et al. Mental and Elemental Nutrients: A Physician's Guide to Nutrition and Health Care.* New Canaan, CT: Keats Publishing, 1975.
Rodale, J. I. *Natural Health, Sugar and the Criminal Mind.* New York: Pyramid Books, 1968.
Royal, Penny C. *Herbally Yours.* Provo, UT: BiWorld Publishers, 1976.

Other Books of Interest

Bricklin, Mark. *The Practical Encyclopedia of Natural Healing.* Emmaus, PA: Rodale Press, 1976.
Cheraskin, Emanuel and Ringsdorf, W. M., Jr. *New Hope for Incurable Diseases.* New York: Exposition Press, 1971.
Coca, Arthur F. *The Pulse Test.* New York: Arco Publishing Company, 1968.
Craig, Sheila. *Tantrums, Toads, and Teddy Bears.* Scottdale, PA: Herald Press, 1979.
Diamond, John. *BK: Behavioral Kinesiology.* New York: Harper & Row, Publishers, 1979.
Ott, John N. *Health and Light: The Effects of Natural and Artificial Light on Man and Other Living Things.* New York: Pocket Books, 1973.
Rapp, Doris J. *Allergies and the Hyperactive Child.* New York: Sovereign Books, 1979.